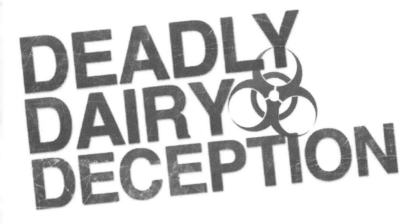

DEADLY DAIRY DECEPTION

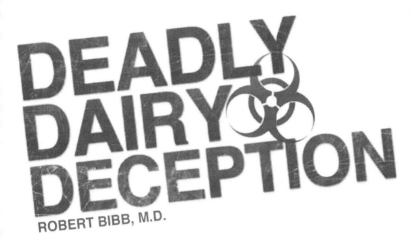

DEADLY DAIRY DECEPTION

ROBERT BIBB, M.D.

TATE PUBLISHING & Enterprises

Published by Tate Publishing & Enterprises, LLC
127 E. Trade Center Terrace | Mustang, Oklahoma 73064 USA
1.888.361.9473 | www.tatepublishing.com

Tate Publishing is committed to excellence in the publishing industry. The company reflects the philosophy established by the founders, based on Psalm 68:11,
"The Lord gave the word and great was the company of those who published it."

Book design copyright © 2010 by Tate Publishing, LLC. All rights reserved.
Cover design by Tyler Evans
Interior design by Jeff Fisher

Published in the United States of America

ISBN: 978-1-61566-773-4
1. Health & Fitness, Diseases, Cancer
2. Health & Fitness, Nutrition
10.02.24

DEDICATION

In memory of my father
Douglas G. Bibb

The only real valuable thing is intuition.

—Albert Einstein

ACKNOWLEDGMENTS

This document would not have been possible, if it were not for the numerous researchers who provided the "food-for-thought" research papers end noted in this book. I must give special thanks to my wife, Barbara, who became an "author's widow" during the preparation of this manuscript. She supported and encouraged me and acted as a sounding board for the numerous thoughts that I had about how to present this information. Barbara is responsible for the title. Special thanks to Mr. Daniel O'Sullivan. This wonderful and brilliant young man is responsible for many of the pieces of artwork in this book. Thanks to Mr. Paul Eastwood. Paul is a professional trainer who prepared Appendix F on protein alternatives other than dairy. A note of thanks to Dr. William Harris; Kathleen McDavid, PhD, and her coauthors; and to Joanna Meadows from Breast

Cancer Research, U.K. All these fine individuals gave me permission to use graphs from their manuscripts and Web sites. I must thank Kris Dempko, who has researched the topic of dairy and the breast cancer thoroughly and pointed me to numerous cited works for my review. I appreciate my friend William Danby M.D., who encouraged and supported my work. I must thank Dr. Richard Tate, the owner of Tate Publishing, and his staff for taking on the task of making this book available to the general public. Special thanks to J. Bode for the fine job of editing my manuscript. Tyler Evans and Jeff Fisher at Tate Publishing who created the cover and interior design of the book that caught your attention. Thank you, Tyler and Jeff.

TABLE OF CONTENTS

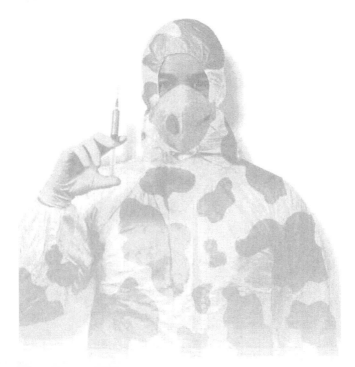

FOREWORD

The most basic tool of all scientists is the "scientific method." This involves formulation of a hypothesis based on previous observations and then testing this hypothesis by experimentation. However, difficulties sometimes arise in applying this approach to systems as complex as organisms—particularly humans with whom the possibilities for experimentation are greatly limited. Because they need to test new theories rigorously, scientists are necessarily slow to change established models. Unfortunately, this conservative approach sometimes leads to a narrow-minded refusal to accept new hypotheses that might challenge ingrained ideas.

Well-known examples include the resistance of physicists (including Einstein) to the quantum theory during the first half of the last century and their reluctance to give up the idea that an ether must be required to transmit electromagnetic waves. Examples in biology include the insistence, prior to Watson and Crick, that proteins, not nucleic acids, carry the genetic information and, more recently, the illusion that once the base sequence of human DNA is known treatment of cancer and other diseases will rapidly become much more effective. Early cancer studies with animals led to the idea that cancer is caused by viruses (e.g. Rous sarcoma, Shope papilloma). But chemicals and radiation were found to cause cancer also, and the idea that cancer is not a transmissible disease became prevalent. Now, we know that viruses (HPV in cervical cancer) and bacteria (H. Pylori in stomach cancer) play roles in the development of some cancers and the complexity of the phenomenon of carcinogenesis is becoming appreciated.

For decades milk and dairy products have been promoted as health foods because of their protein, calcium, and vitamin D contents. Nutritionists suggest that these should compose a significant part of the diets of both children and adults. Here, again, a narrow focus on one aspect of a complex system has been allowed to overshadow any reservations about the simplistic conclusion that "Milk is good for your health." Lactation is induced by pregnancy, which involves large shifts in hormone levels, and these hormones are transmitted in the milk. The data is clear: 1) Milk contains estrogens and other hormones. 2) The likelihood that a woman will develop breast cancer is directly related to the amount of estrogen to which she is exposed during her lifetime. 3) Milk contains the growth factors that can stimulate growth of the newborn. 4) These factors, especially IGF-1, stimulate growth of cancer cells and tumors.

Recent data indicates that in addition to providing exogenous hormones, milk consumption can induce changes in endogenous hormone concentrations including reduction of testosterone levels in men. The complexity of the synthetic pathways of steroid hormones and the interactions among hormones is truly astounding. Even very small changes in the concentrations these hormones can have dramatic effects. Both endocrine systems and the process of carcinogenesis are very far from being understood. To rule out any logical hypothesis about how changes in hormone levels might affect susceptibility to breast or prostate cancer is itself simply naïve.

After a comprehensive examination of the scientific literature, Dr. Bibb became convinced that milk and changes in the way it has been processed since the 1950s have contributed to the epidemic of breast and prostate cancers. He has vigorously encouraged research to test this hypothesis but has encountered resistance from many "scientists" in the areas of nutrition and cancer research. It is exactly this resistance and reluctance to test new hypotheses that has frequently retarded progress in many areas of science. Also, it is unfortunate that in this type of study the direction of scientific enquiry and implementation of the findings are strongly influenced by industrial lobbying and advertising.

Most disturbing is the fact that human lives are at stake. Dr. Bibb has presented a logical hypothesis based on data published in the peer-reviewed literature and based on numerous carefully designed experiments. His ideas are summarized in this book. Refusal to thoroughly explore the possible role dairy products play in cancer is not only biased and unscientific but also unethical.

Dr. Bibb is to be thanked for recognizing the possible role of dairy products in carcinogenesis, suggesting how this risk might be minimized and insisting that this problem be resolved. His hypothesis is based on good data and sound logic. It is essential to the health of both men and women that his hypothesis be accepted as scientifically valid and thoroughly tested experimentally.

—Lyndon L. Larcom
Research Professor of Healthcare Genetics
Clemson University 2009

INTRODUCTION

This book is not about intentional deception on the part of any individual person or industry. It is about inherent properties of dairy products. It is about the proteins and hormones that cows secrete for their calves. Unfortunately, for humans, this secreted liquid we call milk and the products derived from it are deliciously deceptive. They taste good. To many of us, milk and the products, such as cheese and ice cream, made from milk are comfort foods. It is, however, this delicious and comfortable deception that exposes the public to the hormones and proteins that I believe are the cause of the prostate cancer epidemic and likely estrogen receptor positive breast cancer. The processes outlined in this book may also be true for other tissues that contain estrogen and growth factor receptors. It is time for government and private institutions to support the testing of the hypothesis that dairy is the main cause of hormonally sensitive cancers. The information in this book will hopefully inspire those who read it to demand that such research begin. I hope that those with hormonally sensitive tumors would eliminate dairy from their diets. There is greater hope for their survival with such a determination.

I have a personal stake in making the dairy cancer information public. This stake is not driven for personal gain but simply by a deep concern for what I have learned. I want to share this knowledge with all those that have been connected with the disease we call cancer.

My father developed non-Hodgkin's lymphoma when I was in medical school. He was forty-eight. His mother, my grandmother, had died of ovarian cancer when she was in her mid-forties.

My father was always worried that "some cancer gene(s)" existed in his family tree and that he had passed them on to his children. Being the all-knowing medical student, I assured him that there was no connection between the two cancers. I was wrong.

I wrote this book so that others could gain some of the knowledge I have acquired. Discover what I have learned. Discover why I was wrong.

Be Worried; Be Very Worried

It may surprise readers of this book to learn that I am a dermatologist and may further intrigue them as to how I came to write a book about prostate cancer development.

My father's death due to non-Hodgkin's lymphoma at an early age led to my leaving a career in radiation health physics with a major corporation and entering medical school in 1975. I had an expectation that with my chemical engineering background and graduate work in bioenvironmental engineering, I could positively affect an expected tenure as a radiation oncologist. A strong interest in skin disease, during medical school, led me in a different direction.

Most dermatology residencies introduce the budding physician to the mechanisms behind skin cancer development. My residency at the Medical University of South Carolina in Charleston, South Carolina, was exceptional in this regard. The basic mechanisms behind cancer development were a strong interest from then on.

As a dermatologist, I routinely deal with melanoma. As dermatologists, we are taught that there is only one single identifiable factor that is avoidable in reducing the incidence of deadly melanoma skin cancer: ultraviolet light. And as I hope to explain in this book, so it is with the hormonally sensitive tumor, cancer of the prostate gland. I believe that the only single identifiable and preventive measure to prevent prostate cancer and other hormonally sensitive cancers is avoidance of milk and milk-derived products.

Two fortuitous events would capture my intuitive scientific interest and propel me to investigate the prostate cancer-dairy link.

Dr. Daniel Nixon, then at the Medical University of South Carolina, was investigating the benefit of red raspberry consumption on tissue cultures of human cancers. These cultures included prostate cancer tissue. Dr. Nixon's research interested me, and during investigation of his work, I learned that prostate cancer incidence (men per 100,000) had been on an upward slope since the early 1950s. The reason for this rise had resisted any rational explanation.

At a national meeting of dermatologists, almost a decade ago, Dr. William Danby was discussing his work on the relationship of dairy consumption and acne development. I was in the audience listening intently to what he was saying. He related that the dairy industry used to expose milk to ultraviolet light to generate vitamin D and that this process was abandoned in the late 1940s. I knew that this could not be a coincidence. Milk exposure to ultraviolet light stops, and prostate cancer incidence increases!

When I started this project seven years ago, my fellow physicians laughed at the idea that dairy could be behind the epidemic of prostate and breast cancer. I told them specifically that I thought that estrogens are not only involved in the development of breast cancer but prostate cancer also. I entertained this idea with several dairy department professors, who did not specifically say I was wrong but implied that this was the case. I feel vindicated by the plethora of studies indicating that I am correct. I do not believe that it is a question of whether dairy causes breast and prostate cancer but of how it does so.

I have reviewed the literature on the mechanisms of prostate cancer development available for the last two decades and must give credit to the multitude of researchers that provided me with the information you are going to read about. From this literature, I have put forth a cohesive explanation for the development of prostate cancer, which includes the genetic, biochemical, and hormonal interactions that lead to development of this cancer. I will tell you that it is likely that all the hormonally sensitive tumors, such as estrogen-receptor-positive breast cancer, testicular cancer, endometrial, lymphoma, and ovarian cancer may be caused by similar mechanisms related to dairy consumption. I have chosen to concentrate on prostate cancer because this malignancy has the strongest peer-reviewed literature association with ingestion of dairy-related foods.

You will learn not only how the individual, naturally occurring proteins and hormones react within our body but why African-American men have higher rates of prostate and breast cancer compared to their Caucasian counterparts. You will learn why your dairy consumption may affect your children and your grandchildren, and lastly, I will explain why there is hope for the future of dairy and the people that have been affected by its consumption.

Before we begin the factual journey, I must tell you a story. Recently, one busy morning in my office, I was relating the dairy story to one of my patients. He said, "Dr. Bibb, I don't do dairy. I was raised on a dairy farm." After learning all the scientific facts about dairy and the connection to cancer, I can understand his fear. Be worried. Be very worried.

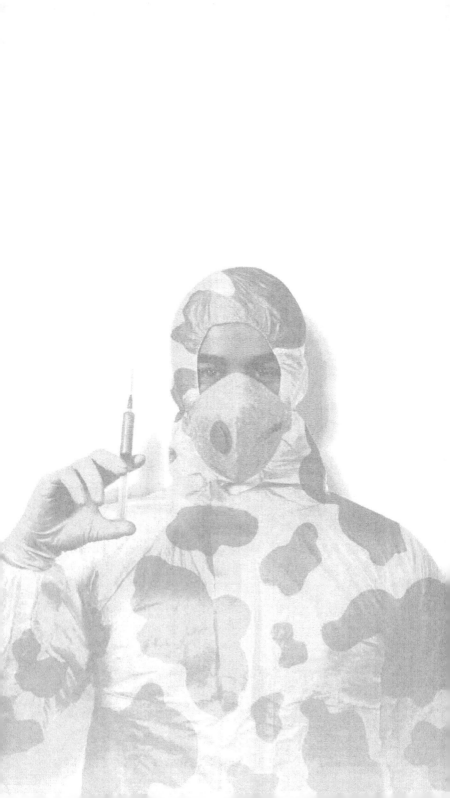

PROSTATE CANCER: THE DISEASE

The prostate gland is part of the male reproductive system and is responsible for producing the fluid called seminal fluid in which is carried the sperm. It sits below the urinary bladder and in front of the rectum. It partially surrounds the urethra (see Figure One).[1] It normally is about the size of a walnut. The individual cells that comprise the gland as a whole consist of the secretory cells imbedded in a fibrous connective tissue known as the *stroma* (See Figure Two). [2] When we use the term *prostate cancer*, it is generally assumed to be an *adenocarcinoma*, which in medical terminology means "a cancer of the secretory cells." The prostate gland is also the gland that produces the so-called antigen (PSA), which is a sugar-connected protein used in detecting and monitoring prostate cancer.

Figure One: The Male-Reproductive Tract[3]

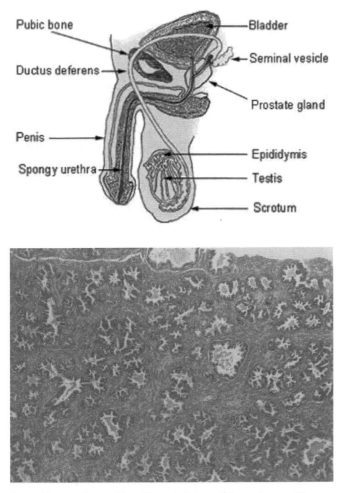

Figure Source: Figure Two: Normal Prostate Tissue. Source: Dreamstime, "Prostatic tissue young human," (2009) http://www.dreamstime.com/royalty-free-stock-photos-pr[4]ostatic-tissue-young-human-image6166778. Reproduced by licensure.[5]

Normal prostate tissue is divided into the fibrous, connective tissue known as the *stroma*, which is the solid material and the secretory cells that line the hollow cavities, or ducts, as illustrated in Figure Two. The secretory cells are the cells that change into malignant cells resulting in adenocarcinoma, or prostate cancer.

Cancer for the most part is a "dance of the genes." What I mean by this is that there are genes that prevent cells from dying, and there are genes that cause cells to die. If a gene that causes a cell to die becomes defective, or conversely a gene that keeps a cell from dying becomes defective, then a cell can become immortal and pass its inability to die on to its daughter cells and so on. You then have a group of cells that does not die. You have now developed a cancer. And so it is with prostate cancer. One specific gene found to be defective in prostate cancer is the so-called p53 gene. It causes cells to die and has been found to be defective in many cancers, including prostate.

In normal cell division the effect of the p53 gene is to cause a natural cell death in either aged or defective cells. This is illustrated in Figure Three.[6]

Figure Three[7]: Normal p53—mediated-cell death.

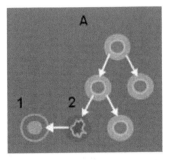

When a cell divides as controlled by a normal p53 gene, a healthy colony of cells proliferates (A). When a cell becomes affected with an abnormality (2), a healthy p53 gene will cause it to die (1).

In prostate cells that have become cancerous because of a defect in the p53 gene and/or other genes that control cell death, the cells do not die, and they pass this inability to die on to daughter cells and so on, down the line until a tumor has developed. This is illustrated in Figure Four.[8]

Figure Four[9]: Defective p53 and cancer colony.

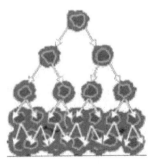

If a cell contains a defective p53 gene and/or other suppressor gene defects, a cancerous colony develops.

The prostate cells and, therefore, the prostate gland itself are under the influence of many hormones and proteins. The hormones and proteins provide their effect by attaching to the myriad of receptors that have been so far identified. These receptors, hormones, and proteins play an important role in determining the health of the prostate gland and whether a man will develop cancer from an abnormal stimulation of the receptors by the proteins and hormones.

These hormones and proteins are powerful agents, and their stimulation acts through what is known as the secondary messenger system. It is like a bowling ball striking the number one pin in such a way to affect all the pins. In this way a single molecule of a protein or hormone can magnify the end effect by a hundred, a thousand, or even more.

The prostate gland can be influenced by hormones or proteins given orally or by injection. It is also influenced by endogenous hormones made by glands distant to it, such as those manufactured by the pituitary, testes, and adrenal glands. These glands release their hormones directly into the bloodstream. This is called endocrine secretion.

The prostate cells lining the ducts can be influenced by cells adjacent to them that secrete proteins and hormones. An example would be the stromal cells (connective tissue) producing proteins and hormones that affect the duct cells. This is known as *paracrine secretion*. Even the prostate cells themselves can produce proteins or hormones that affect the cell type that produced them. This is known as *autocrine secretion*.

Autocrine secretion is thought to play an important role in self-stimulating the growth of prostate and breast cells, once they have become malignant.[10] Figures Five, Six, and Seven are illustrative of these processes.

Figure Five[11]: Endocrine effects on adrenal, testes, and prostate glands.

Endocrine Effects On the Prostate Gland

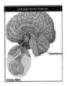

Hypothalamus causes pituitary gland to release leutinizing hormone

Leutinizing hormone causes testes to release testosterone

ACTH causes adrenal gland to release androstenedione, DHEA, and DHEA-Sulfate

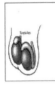

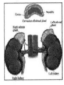

Testosterone influences the prostate

Adrenal gland hormones are converted to make hormones in the prostate

Figure Six[12]: Paracrine stimulation

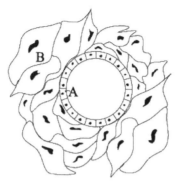

Paracrine secretion occurs when stroma cells (B) produce hormones, which stimulate duct cells (A).

Figure Seven[13]: Autocrine Stimulation

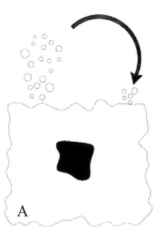

Prostatee pithelial cell (A) releases hormones and proteins that restimulate the same type of cells.]

The suspicion that a man has developed prostate cancer is made in a variety of ways. A man can present with difficulty urinating, blood in his urine, pain in the groin region, and a lump or nodule can be felt on the prostate gland during digital rectal exam. Another suspicion could be that the prostate-specific antigen blood test is rising rapidly enough to suspect that cancer has developed. If prostate cancer suspicion is strong enough, a series of prostate needle biopsies may be obtained. An actual example of the mapping done during these needle biopsies is presented in Figure Eight.[14] Figure Eight is a copy of a biopsy report on an actual patient with cancer of the prostate before dairy abstinence.

Figure Eight[15]: Patient H.W. abnormal prostate biopsy prior to dairy-free diet

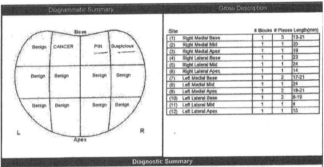

Site		# Blocks	# Pieces	Length(mm)
(1)	Right Medial Base	1	3	13-21
(2)	Right Medial Mid	1	1	20
(3)	Right Medial Apex	1	1	19
(4)	Right Lateral Base	1	1	23
(5)	Right Lateral Mid	1	1	24
(6)	Right Lateral Apex	1	1	14
(7)	Left Medial Base	1	2	17-21
(8)	Left Medial Mid	1	1	24
(9)	Left Medial Apex	1	2	19-21
(10)	Left Lateral Base	1	2	8-19
(11)	Left Lateral Mid	1	1	4
(12)	Left Lateral Apex	1	1	15

Diagnostic Summary
Adenocarcinoma, Gleason score 6 (3+3). Tumor involves the left side of the prostate.

Note: PIN is an abbreviation for prostate intraepithelial neoplasia. PIN is the designation given to the very early form of prostate cancer.

Figure Nine[16]: Patient H.W. normal prostate biopsy after one year on a dairy-free diet

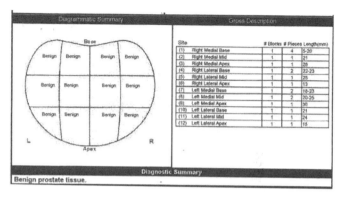

Site	# Blocks	# Pieces	Length(mm)
(1) Right Medial Base	1	4	5-20
(2) Right Medial Mid	1	1	21
(3) Right Medial Apex	1	1	28
(4) Right Lateral Base	1	2	22-23
(5) Right Lateral Mid	1	1	25
(6) Right Lateral Apex	1	1	13
(7) Left Medial Base	1	2	18-23
(8) Left Medial Mid	1	2	20-25
(9) Left Medial Apex	1	1	30
(10) Left Lateral Base	1	1	21
(11) Left Lateral Mid	1	1	24
(12) Left Lateral Apex	1	1	16

Diagnostic Summary

Benign prostate tissue.

Note: Patient spared a radical prostatectomy.

If cancer is found in a biopsy, a so-called Gleason score is determined for that particular tumor.

The Gleason score is determined by how far from normal the malignant cells appear under the microscope. Malignant cells are graded on the basis of what is called *differentiation*. A well-differentiated, prostate cancer cell is close to the appearance of that of a normal prostate cell. A poorly-differentiated prostate cancer cell differs markedly from the normal cell. A scale has been developed to grade prostate cancer cells from well differentiated (1 on the scale) to poorly differentiated (5 on the scale) and is coded in numbers 1–5. (See the Gleason grading scale in Figure Ten.)[17]

Figure Ten[18]: Gleason score

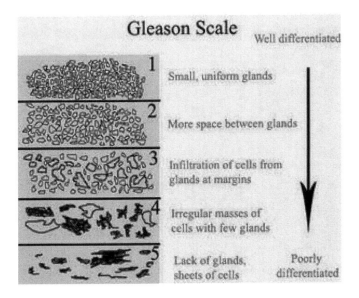

The so-called Gleason score is the sum of the most common cell type plus the second most common cell type and would have a maximum of ten. The Gleason score is used by physicians to guide treatment options and can be a measure of long-term survival predictability.

What You Should Have Learned From This Chapter:

1. The p53 gene is a very important gene in determining whether the prostate gland becomes malignant.

2. The only way to determine whether a man has prostate cancer is with a biopsy procedure.

3. The Gleason score is determined by adding the two most common cell type scores.

4. The Gleason score will determine what is recommended next in treatment options.

PROSTATE CANCER: THE STATISTICS

Statistical data can be useful information in that it can provide us data to look at trends in disease processes. I have provided in this chapter some of the more shocking data to give the reader an idea about how prevalent this disease we call prostate cancer really is. This information tells us that prostate cancer incidence is increasing to epidemic proportions. Incidence is defined as the number of people per 100,000 or in our case the number of men with prostate cancer per 100,000 men in any given population.

Prostate cancer is the number one cancer affecting men in the United States. From 720,280 cases of cancer reported in 2006, 33 percent were prostate cancer.

Table One: Percent Cancer Reported for Men in 2006.[2]

PROSTATE	**33%**
Lung and Bronchus	13%
Colon and Rectum	11%
Urinary Bladder	6%
Melanoma	5%
Lymphoma	4%
Kidney	3%
Oral	3%
Leukemia	3%
Pancreas	2%
All Other	22%

Note: From American Cancer Society, 2006.[3]

The age adjusted incidence (people per 100,000) of prostate cancer in the U.S. has risen 266 percent between the years 1950 and 1992.[2] While other cancer rates have decreased, prostate cancer rates have climbed.

Figure One: Cancer incidence rates for men, 1975–2002

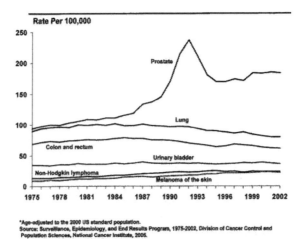

Age-adjusted to the 2000 US standard population.
Source: Surveillance, Epidemiology, and End Results Program, 1975-2002, Division of Cancer Control and Population Sciences, National Cancer Institute, 2005.

Note: The sudden spike in incidence represents cancers that were discovered by the newly emerging PSA test in 1986. The baseline curve continues upward on the same slope, after the test is established.

The steep increases in incidence are not solely observed in the U.S. alone but are seen in other Western cultures as well. The following incidence curves demonstrate this point.

☠

Figure Two: Standardized (European) incidence and mortality rates prostate cancer, G.B., 1975–2002.

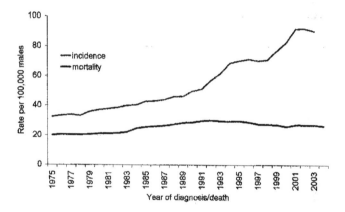

Figure Two: Reproduced by permission from: http://info.cancerresearchuk.org/cancerstats/types/prostate/incidence/

Figure Three: Prostate cancer incidence and mortality rates, Canada and United States

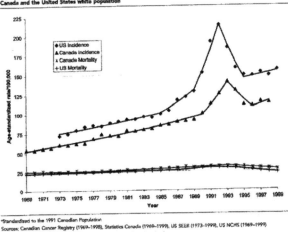

Figure 1. Age-standardized* prostate cancer incidence and mortality rates, Canada and the United States white population

*Standardized to the 1991 Canadian Population
Sources: Canadian Cancer Registry (1969–1998), Statistics Canada (1969–1999), US SEER (1973–1999), US NCHS (1969–1999)
NOTE: Points represent observed rates; lines represent joinpoint regression lines.

Figure Three: Reproduced by permission from: Kathleen McDavid, PhD, MPH; Judy Lee, MA; John P. Fulton, PhD; Jon Tonita, MSc; and Trevor D. Thompson,"Cancer Prostate Incidence and Mortali-tyRates and Trends in the United States and Canada," Public Health Rep. 119 (2004):174–86. http://www.ncbi.nlm.nih.gov/pmc/articles/PMC1497609/

If one looks at the international prostate cancer incidence rates presented for the time periods of 1988–1992 and 1993–1997, it can generally be appreciated that there is a drift upward of the incidence in each country; however, the rates remain low in countries that have not developed significant Western lifestyles.

Table Two: Prostate cancer international incidence rates:

COUNTRY	1988-1992	1993-1997
USA	119.0	146.4
CANADA	65.0	80.2
SWEDEN	55.0	63.0
SWITZERLAND	49.0	52.4
NORWAY	48.0	60.9
FRANCE	44.0	53.6
FINLAND	41.0	62.8
GERMANY	36.0	49.4
DENMARK	31.0	29.9
ENGLAND & WALES	28.0	39.6
COSTA RICA	27.0	33.1
ITALY	12.0	20.1
SINGAPORE	10.0	14.1
JAPAN	9.0	12.7
INDIA	8.0	7.4
HONG KONG	8.0	8.6
CHINA	2.0	3.0

Sources: 1. Parkin, D.M., Whalen, S.L., Ferlay, J., and Young, J, eds. (1997) Cancer Incidence in Five Continents, Vol. Vll. IARC Scientific Publications No. 143 Lyon IARC and 2. Parkin, D.M., Whalen, S.L., Ferlay, J., Teppo, L. and Thomas, D.B. eds, (2003) Cancer Incidence in Five Continents, Vol. Vlll, IARC Scientific Publications N0.155. Lyon IARC.

Not only is the incidence of prostate cancer increasing worldwide, but the average age at which men living in Western cultures develop this disease is dropping. If we look at the data collected in the U.S. in the interval 1975–2004, this alarming trend can be seen:

Table Three: The prostate cancer incidence rates for African-American men and white men in the age category 20–54 over time.

YEAR	BLACK MEN	WHITE MEN
1975	8	4
1980	7	5
1985	10	5
1990	12	7
1995	43	16
2000	57	25

Source: SEER Statistical Data Base, U.S. Government, "Age Adjusted Incidence Rates by Race for Prostate Cancer, Ages 20–54 Males SEER 9 Registries for 1975–2004. Age Adjusted to the 2000 Std. Population." (2008) http://seer.cancer.gov/csr/1975_2004/results_merged/topic_annualrates.pdf.

There have been a number of published studies looking at autopsy specimens of the prostate glands from men who have died from causes other than cancer. Such deaths included gunshot wounds, automobile accidents, and other miscellaneous accidental causes of death. These studies looked at the incidence rates of early lesions of developing prostate cancer known as *prostate intraepithelial neoplasia* (PIN). These autopsy findings have consistently found PIN in men in their early thirties and forties. The younger age groups with PIN were typically of African-American ethnicity. This data is summarized in Table Four.

Table Four: Early prostate cancer findings (PIN) by autopsy, ethnic group, and age from various countries.

AUTHOR(S)	FINDINGS OR CONCLUSIONS
Yatani R.., et al. Japan 1988[3]	Although age groups not identified, 22.5% of 576 specimens in 1965-1979 with PIN compared to 34.6% of specimens with PIN from 660 men in 1982-1986.
Sakr WA., et al. USA 1995[4]	218 Afro-American men (AA) and 152 © Caucasian men above age 20 studied and categorized by % and decade of life. For AA 18, 31, 69, 78, 86% in their 4, 5, 6, 7, 8th decades of life vs 14, 21, 38, 50, 63% in 4, 5, 6, 7, 8th decades of life for C.
Sánchez CM., et al. 2001 Spain[5]	% PIN averages were 7.1, 14.7, 28.5, 33.3, 45.4, and 51.8 in the 4th, 5th, 6th, 7th and 8th decades respectively. (these were Caucasian Spaniards)
Soos G., et al., Hungary 2005[6]	In the age group 81-95, 86.6% had PIN with PIN being detected as early as the 3rd decade of life.
Dewailly E., et al., Canada 2003[7]	All deaths in Greenland males that occurred between 1990-1994 were autopsied with only one case of invasive prostate cancer found. No early cases of prostate cancer were noted.

Several points are worth noting from the data summarized in Table Four.

1. The cases pointed out in Table Four were early prostate cancers detected by autopsy only. For the most part, these men did not have cancer that was yet detected by any clinical evaluation, such as a laboratory test or physical abnormality. In other words, these men did not know they had cancer yet.

2. African-American men had higher over-all rates of undetected prostate cancer and on the average had developed their cancer almost a decade before their Caucasian counterparts.

3. Inuit men (Greenland men) seem protected against prostate cancer. The conclusion of the authors of this paper was that the high intake of omega-3 in the Inuit diet was the protective factor against prostate cancer.[8] The protective effect of omega-3 fats has been disputed by a systematic review of the literature by MacLean.[9] With this information in mind, the other factor that may have played a more significant role is that the Inuit do not consume dairy products.

It would appear that from the autopsy evidence that the incidence of prostate cancer is much higher than is obvious because the epidemiologic data only include the number of men who have actually been reported to have obvious prostate cancer.

What You Should Have Learned From This Chapter

1. Prostate cancer incidence is increasing worldwide.

2. Prostate cancer incidence is highest in Western cultures.

3. The age at which men get obvious prostate cancer is dropping.

4. Autopsy studies have revealed that a significant percentage of men have prostate cancer at an early age, and it is not yet detected.

5. Autopsy studies reveal that African-American men develop prostate cancer almost a decade earlier than their Caucasian counterparts.

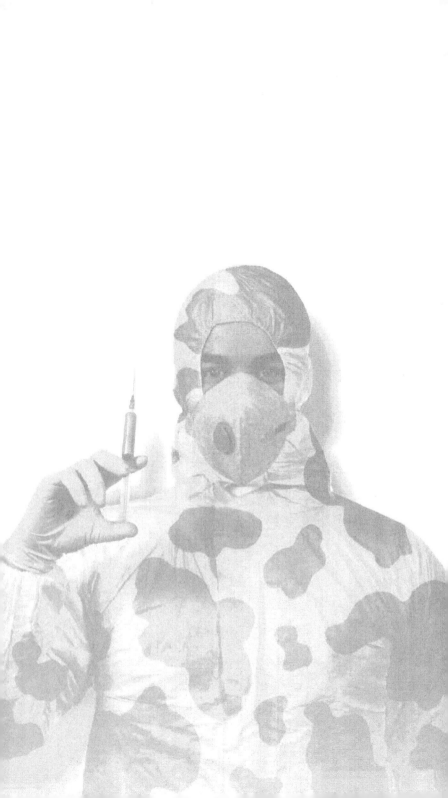

FOOD ASSOCIATION STUDIES

Many food association studies have been performed over the years trying to link certain dietary habits to certain cancers. There are generally two types of studies that are used to develop risk associations with diet. These are called case-controlled studies and cohort studies.

Case-controlled studies compare diets of individuals with cancer to those who do not have cancer. An attempt is made to match the individuals for age and other similar characteristics. The dietary information is determined by extensive questioning and relies on dietary habit recall. These studies are limited because they rely on memory recall, and they are confounded with the difficulty of trying to sort out what foods actually have dairy derivatives in them. We, retrospectively, also know that foods that may have dairy derivatives in them may not have been included in the questioning. These studies could significantly underestimate the amount of dairy consumed because patients may not have been aware that they were consuming dairy-containing foods, such as those incorporating whey and casein. In essence, case-controlled studies can be manipulated by the type of questions asked. Case-controlled studies are not as accurate as cohort studies.

Cohort studies look at groups of individuals over time, collect dietary information, and then look at the cases of a particular cancer that has developed. Cohort studies by design more accurately reflect the association of a diet with a particular cancer because the cohort studies compare groups of individuals who are basically the same except for one main difference. In this book it would be comparing individuals consuming little or no dairy to individuals who consumed dairy. This important fact should be kept in mind. Shortly before my book was published, two case-controlled studies were reported that claimed that there was a poor association with dairy consumption and prostate cancer. Hmm.

Now let us take a look at the burden of peer-reviewed literature linking dairy consumption with a higher risk of prostate cancer. I am going to review these studies in chronological order.

Talamini and associates in 1986 looked at 166 patients with confirmed prostate cancer and compared them to 202 patients without prostate cancer in a case-controlled study. This study revealed that moderately overweight men had a greater risk of prostate cancer, as did cases that reported frequent consumption of milk.

From the prestigious Roswell Park Memorial Institute in Buffalo, New York in a case-controlled study in 1986, Mettlin and fellow researchers found that men with high-fat milk consumption and a habit of drinking three or more glasses of whole milk daily had 1.9 and 2.5 times greater risk of developing prostate cancer respectively.[2]

From another Italian study in 1991, LaVecchia and his associates looked at increasing levels of milk consumption and found a "significant trend" of increasing cases of prostate cancer associated with increased consumption of milk.[3]

From Sweden in 1998, Chan and his fellow laboratory collaborators looked at 526 cases of prostate cancer and compared them to 536 controls and found that: "High consumption of dairy products was associated with a 50 percent increased risk of developing prostate cancer."[4]

Jumping back to the NASA facility at Langley Research Center in Virginia in 1999, Grant used a multifactorial, statistical approach, looked at 41 countries, and concluded that the nonfat portion of milk had the highest association with prostate cancer, as was found in other reviewed cohort studies.[5] A multifactorial study tries to remove confounding factors that might influence the interpretation.

From the year 2000 and the country that gave us pizza (Italy), Bosetti and his team looked at a case-controlled study conducted in Athens, Greece, which found that dairy and butter consumption were positively associated with risk of prostate cancer.[6]

From Harvard in 2002, Chan and fellow authors investigated the association between dairy products and calcium intakes and prostate cancer risk in the Physicians' Health Study, a cohort of male US physicians, and found:

> Compared with men consuming ≤150 mg Ca/d from dairy products, men consuming ˃ 600 mg/d had a 32 percent higher risk of prostate cancer (95 percent CI: 1.08, 1.63).[7] (Ca/d means Calcium per day. This essentially means dairy products consumed per day.)

Conclusions: This Harvard investigation supports the hypothesis that dairy products and calcium are associated with *greater risk of prostate cancer.*[8]

From a 2004 Japanese statistical analysis of eleven available U.S. cohort studies, it was concluded that there is a positive association between milk consumption and prostate cancer.[9]

From a large, case-controlled study in Italy in 2004, Bosetti and his colleagues reported on 1,294 men studied over the years 1991–2002. They reported a significant trend of increasing risk for prostate cancer with more frequent consumption of milk and dairy products.[10]

From a French study in 2006, Keese and fellow authors reported that their data review supported the following hypothesis:

> … that dairy products have a harmful effect with respect to the risk of prostate cancer, largely related to Ca content. The higher risk of prostate cancer

with linear increasing yoghurt consumption seems to be independent of Ca and may be related to some other component.[11]

Hmm, "other components," huh? These other components will be discussed in the following chapters.

From the Johns Hopkins Bloomberg School of Public Health in 2007, Rohrmann and fellow authors reported on 3,892 men thirty-five-plus years of age that completed a food survey study. The subsequent incidence of prostate cancer was ascertained for the group. The authors reported that there was a positive association with dairy intake but not calcium consumption with increased risk of prostate cancer.[12]

And from up north with the reindeer, a study from 2007 in Finland found total dietary intake of dairy was associated with an increased risk for prostate cancer.[13]

And finally, the latest and greatest study in 2008 from Japan has revealed the following information. In a prospective cohort study of over 43,000 Japanese men in the age group 45–74 followed for 7.5 years, it was revealed that[14]:

> …dairy products were associated with a dose-dependent increase in the risk of prostate cancer. The relative risks (95 percent confidence intervals) comparing the highest with the lowest quartiles of total dairy products, milk, and yogurt were 1.63 (1.14–2.32), 1.53 (1.07–2.19), and 1.52 (1.10–2.12).[15]

The authors went on to state: "In summary, we found that the intake of dairy products was associated with an increased risk of prostate cancer."[16]

Study after study has found an increased risk of prostate cancer associated with dairy consumption. So if I do not have you running to empty most of your refrigerator into the garbage, read on! The indictment of dairy continues.

It would make sense that if increasing dairy consumption is associated with increased risk of prostate cancer then we might be able to look at the incidence (people per 100,000 of the population) of hormonally sensitive tumors in different countries and see if we can associate it with dairy consumption. It would be very interesting if we knew the *per-capita consumption* ("pounds per person") of dairy for these countries and could plot out incidence versus per-capita consumption. This graph might be able to tell us something about the relationship between the consumption of dairy products and any relationship to certain cancers.

There is a mathematical technique that uses certain computer programs to determine the graph of the consumption of dairy products and their relationship to cancer. If the computer program recognizes a straight line, then a strong association exists. This technique can tell us if a linear (direct correlation) exists between dairy consumption and incidence of prostate cancer and other cancers by looking at something called a *P value*. If a P value is small (i.e., less than 1), then a very strong association exists.

As you would probably guess, these studies have been done. William Harris, MD, reports on these linear, or straight-line, associations. Dr. Harris has conveniently drawn by computer analysis the straight-line associations that exist between dairy consumption and various cancers. I have included the graphs for ovarian and prostate cancer in this section. Dr. Harris has also plotted out other interesting associations between dairy consumption and cancer.[17] Look at these other associations in the appendix D. Remember these associations because they will be discussed later.

Figure One: Ovarian cancer incidence by country versus animal source calcium.[18]

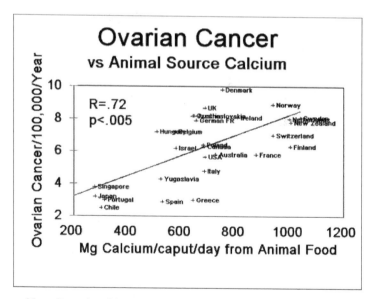

Note: Reproduced by permission. Harris, W. M.D., "Cancer and the Vegetarian Diet" (1999). http://www.vegsource.com/harris/cancer_vegdiet.htm.[19] (The mg. of calcium are basically from dairy.)

The most significant characteristic about the curve in Figure One is that *it is a straight line!* This means that there is a direct correlation with dairy intake and incidence of ovarian cancer.

Figure Two: Prostate cancer by country versus animal source calcium.[19]

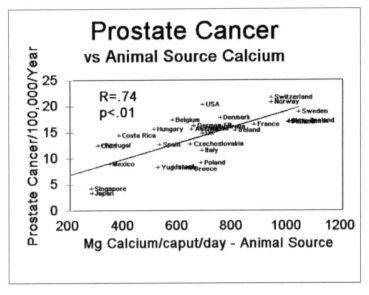

(The mg. of calcium are basically from dairy.)

Note: Reproduced by permission. Harris, W. M.D., "Cancer and the Vegetarian Diet"(1999). http://www.vegsource.com/harris/cancer_vegdiet.htm (accessed Feb. 8, 2008).20

Again, you should note that we have a graph consisting of a straight line with a very small P value. Remember a small P value means a strong association exists. *Dairy consumption and prostate cancer incidence are strongly associated!*

I would hope that the various reports have convinced you that dairy is likely the main cause of hormonally sensitive cancers, such as prostate and breast cancer. But why would this be the case? I will answer this question and hopefully all your questions in the remaining chapters.

What You Should Have Learned From This Chapter:

1. Dairy consumption has been strongly associated with an increased risk of prostate cancer.

2. The risk of prostate cancer found in these studies cited may be greater than calculated because of failure to include products that have unobvious dairy-related proteins and hormones such as whey and casein.

3. There is a direct correlation between dairy consumption and prostate cancer incidence when numerous countries are studied.

4. There is a direct correlation between dairy consumption and ovarian cancer incidence when numerous countries are studied.

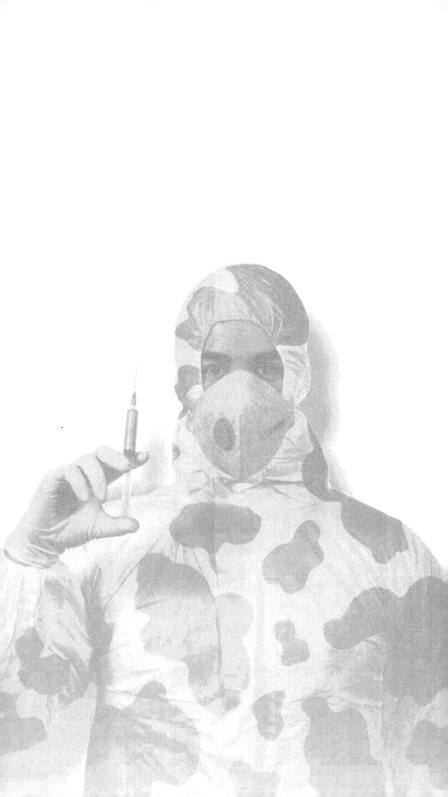

HARRY STEENBOCK
AND THE
ANTIRACHITIC
MACHINE

At the conclusion of a lecture given by Dr. William Danby on his work associating dairy consumption with acne, my intuitive scientific interest was piqued. I knew I had to learn more about the exposure of milk to ultraviolet light.

The story actually begins in 1924 when Professor Harry Steenbock, a biochemist at the University of Wisconsin, discovered a method of activating vitamin D in certain foods. Professor Steenbock had been working on ways to effectively treat rickets, which is caused by a nutritional deficiency of vitamin D. Rickets was a disease of epidemic proportions during the early 1900s in inner-city children. The lack of exposure to ultraviolet light, while living in an inner-city, led to the epidemic. The disease was then known as *rachitis* and resulted in weakened and deformed bones secondary to lack of the vitamin.

Steenbock learned that if cow's milk was exposed to certain wavelengths of ultraviolet light, ergosterol in milk would spontaneously form vitamin D. The ergosterol is a steroid-like compound naturally occurring in plants. When cows eat plants, they secrete ergosterol in their milk. Dr. Steenbock took advantage of this secretion and converted the ergosterol to vitamin D, using his newly discovered technique.[2] (See Figure One.)[3] The consumption of milk and milk-derived products became a convenient and palatable way of administering vitamin D. Cod-liver oil was the nasty alternative at this time.

Figure One: Conversion of ergosterol to vitamin D2 by ultraviolet light.[4]

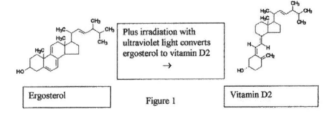

Figure 1

Professor Steenbock went on to develop a method of exposing milk to ultraviolet light during the dairy-processing procedure. The technique used a quartz lamp capable of emitting ultraviolet rays. This process did not significantly slow down the flow of milk through the processing facilities. The process was performed in a nitrogen gas-rich environment to reduce flavor changes caused by oxygen interaction with chemicals existing in the milk.[5] By 1935 thirty-five million people a year consumed milk treated by this process.[6]

Professor Steenbock received a patent for this process in 1928 and donated the proceeds from royalties earned on this patent to an organization he founded at the University of Wisconsin. At the time the patent was granted, the Quaker Oats Company offered Dr. Steenbock one million dollars for the rights to use it. Dr. Steenbock instead licensed the technology to this company and donated the proceeds as described above.[7]

The vitamin D formed by his process was named Viosterol.[8] Harry Steenbock had saved the world from rachitis (Rickets). The process of exposure of milk to ultraviolet light continued until the mid-1940s and was abandoned by the late 1940s, when it became more economical to commercially manufacture vitamin D and add it to the milk.

**Figure Two: Dr. Steenbock and His
Antirachitic Machine.**[9]

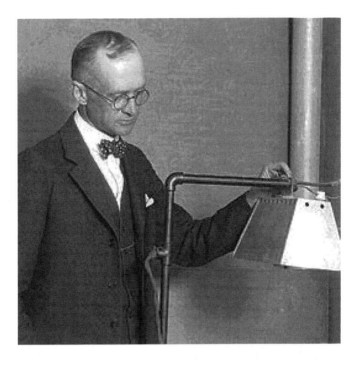

Vitamin D is a hormone. Many hormones are produced from human consumption of cholesterol. The function of a hormone is to control certain other processes in our body. An example of such a process is how the hormone testosterone causes a boy to develop into a man. Hormones can have dramatic consequences on human health. These consequences can be positive and negative. Hormones act through what are known as *secondary messenger systems*. Minute quantities of a hormone can have their action magnified many times through this system. Imagine a bowling ball as the hormone molecule. When this ball strikes the number one pin in just the right manner, all the pins in the group can be affected. This is a simplistic but important principle on how powerful very small amounts of hormones can affect their end organ. A good example would be how the testes grow during puberty or how your son seems to sprout one foot in a year under the influence of testosterone.

Dr. Harry Steenbock took advantage of using ultraviolet light to convert one hormone into another. We should be forever grateful to this brilliant man for curing rickets in his lifetime. Dr. Steenbock also saved many other people from prostate and other hormonally sensitive cancers in ways he never had a chance to appreciate. A segment of the patent number 1,680,818—granted to Dr. Harry Steenbock in 1928—is featured in Figure Three.[10]

Figure Three: Segment of the Steenbock patent.[11]

Patented Aug. 14, 1928.   1,680,818

UNITED STATES PATENT OFFICE.

HARRY STEENBOCK, OF MADISON, WISCONSIN, ASSIGNOR TO WISCONSIN ALUMNI RESEARCH FOUNDATION, A CORPORATION.

ANTIRACHITIC PRODUCT AND PROCESS.

No Drawing.   Application filed June 30, 1924. Serial No. 723,171.

This invention relates particularly to a method of preparing antirachitic products of edible character, such as foods and medicines, and to the products obtained by such method of treatment.

The process is effected by subjecting edible substances to the action of rays of the region of the ultra violet rays of the spectrum in such manner as to effect the antirachitic activation, care being taken to avoid the destruction of the antirachitic principle after it has been imparted. The sterilization of water by means of ultra violet rays is known. Also, it has been proposed to sterilize milk by means of ultra violet rays, but the treatment given to the milk to effect sterilization has also had the effect of spoiling the taste and otherwise injuring the milk, and thus this method of sterilization has failed to come into commercial use. Also, it has been proposed to employ X-rays, or Roentgen rays, to effect sterilization. These rays are not suited to the present purpose, however.

function is to preserve the normal deposition of calcium salts in the bones, thus preventing rachitis, or the disease commonly known as rickets. Again, there is supposed to exist a substance known as factor X, which is concerned with the maintenance of the function of reproduction.

The present invention is particularly concerned with the so-called antirachitic vitamin, but it is to be observed that it is possible to prepare food stuffs for man, and feeds for animals, possessing the properties, or principle, of two or more of the so-called vitamins. The same is true with respect to medicines.

It has long been known that cod liver oil is an excellent therapeutic agent for the prevention and cure of rickets in children. This product, known on the market as cod liver oil, is produced from the livers of certain fishes, most notably the cod fish. However, cod liver oil is not well adapted for use in foods, or as medicine, because of its highly objectionable odor and taste.

In a seminal scientific paper published in 1992 and entitled "Hormones and Growth Factors in Milk," Clark E. Grosvenor and others identified fifty-four bioactive proteins and hormones in milk. These included estradiol, estriol, progesterone, and testosterone, which are hormones. He additionally discovered the powerful hormone-like protein known as insulin-like growth factor-1 (IGF-1).[12] Cow's milk is much like human milk, with both containing PSA (prostate specific antigen) the identical estrogen hormones and insulin-like growth factor one.

Proteins are comprised of linked amino acids. Proteins build, among other things, muscle. This is why you find them sold in different protein drinks in the bodybuilding gyms and health food stores. Proteins remain active in our body when maintained in a structure similar to a coiled snake. They are held in this configuration by interconnecting bonds between sulfur atoms. These bonds are sensitive to ultraviolet light and can be inactivated by exposure to certain wavelengths of this light. The proteins become unfolded when the sulfur-sulfur bonds (disulfide bonds) are broken. When unfolded, the proteins become biologically inactive. This process of breaking disulfide bonds in proteins is called *denaturing*. You are actually familiar with this process of denaturing without knowing it. When you poach an egg and the slippery portion turns white, you have denatured the proteins in it with heat. Another example is the gelatin that forms when you roast a turkey and then put it in the refrigerator overnight. The gelatin that forms is denatured protein. Using ultraviolet light to denature proteins is just a way of using another form of energy to accomplish the same process.

Most water-soluble proteins and most conjugated (connected to proteins) hormones in milk circulate in the liquid (water) portion of the milk. The process of denaturing a protein, such as insulin-like growth factor-1, is illustrated in Figures Four and Five.[13, 14] Ultraviolet light is used as the energy source to denature the protein.

In Figure Four, a protein is folded on itself by a sulfur-sulfur bond. In this configuration, the protein is active. Inside the body, it can exert its biochemical influence.

Figure Four: Folded protein.[15]

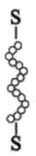

If an ultraviolet light source irradiates (shines) on the protein, it can break the sulfur-sulfur bonds (disulfide bonds), and the protein unfolds and becomes biologically inactive (denatured). It no longer looks or acts like a raw egg. This is illustrated in Figure Five[16]:

Figure Five: Ultraviolet light denaturing a protein.[17]

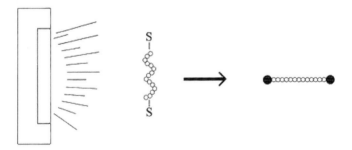

Figure Five[18]: Ultraviolet light strikes a protein, and the protein unfolds and becomes inactive.

Hormones do not contain sulfur-sulfur bonds but can be bound to proteins that do have this link. Hormones can be modified by exposure to ultraviolet light, as Dr. Steenbock had proved with his ultraviolet light treatment of milk. Hormones are generally fat-soluble and would be contained in the fat (lipid) portion of the milk.

In the chapter Prostate Cancer: The Statistics, I outlined the statistical information from the U.S. government, and from this information, it is learned that the incidence slope for prostate cancer strikes the x-axis at zero (zero incidence) in the late 1940s or early 1950s. This is not likely a coincidence. In other words, there was likely very little or no prostate cancer prior to the late 40s or early 50s.

In an experiment by Dr. Lyndom Larcom, tissue cultures of human breast cancer grew rapidly on exposure to commercial milk from the grocery store shelf. This experiment was repeated after the milk was exposed to UV light, and the stimulatory effect had vanished![19]

Let us look again at the incidence of prostate cancer over time. We have good data for incidence back to around 1975 but no readily available data prior to then. This is because this data was not collected in a consistent manner prior to 1975.

Figure Six: SEER incidence rates of
cancer for men 1975–2002.

Rate Per 100,000

*Age-adjusted to the 2000 US standard population.
Source: Surveillance, Epidemiology, and End Results Program, 1975-2002, Division of Cancer Control and
Population Sciences, National Cancer Institute, 2005.

If the incidence curve is extrapolated using the best line to fit the incidence curve for prostate cancer and ignoring the date between 1986 and 1995 (this data is skewed because of the introduction of the PSA test), then the incidence curve will hit the zero incidence line at around 1944. We know that there never was a zero incidence for prostate cancer, but the death rate for prostate cancer has remained reasonably constant over the last fifty years. This rate is roughly twenty-five men per one thousand. If we assume that sixty years ago most men who got prostate cancer died from it, then incidence will roughly equal the death rate. If we extrapolate our graph to this level of incidence, our prostate cancer incidence line strikes twenty-five at around the year 1955 (see Appendix E). If we split the difference between the years 1944 and 1955, then prostate cancer incidence would start to climb around the year 1950. It would seem more than coincidence that the dairy industry abandons milk exposure to ultraviolet light around this time period and prostate and breast cancer incidence starts to increase. A plausible explanation is that proteins including IGF-1 were denatured (inactivated) by the light prior to 1950 and then available as active proteins after 1950 when UV light treatment had been abandoned. This plausible explanation may be borne out by what was observed in Dr. Larcom's experiment.[20] In other words, it is very possible that the dairy industry's use of ultraviolet light made the milk safer to drink prior to 1948 by knocking out the proteins that, I believe, are the major cause of breast and prostate cancer. If I am right about IGF-1 in dairy being one of the major players in prostate cancer, then its destruction with ultraviolet light during the 1920s, 1930s, and 1940s would have dramatically prevented this and other cancers from developing.

Let me take you through the information about IGF-1 and the hormones and proteins in the milk that you are pouring on your cereal in the morning.

What You Should Have Learned From This Chapter:

1. Cow's milk naturally contains estrogens (female hormones), androgens (male hormones), insulin-like growth factor-1, and prostate specific antigen (PSA). Cow's milk is very similar to human milk. With this thought in mind, humans are the only mammals that do not wean their young from the effect of consuming milk.

2. Ultraviolet light probably inactivated certain factors in milk during its use during the 1920s, 1930s, and 1940s.

3. The ultraviolet light treatment process was phased out during the late 1940s because it became less expensive to manufacture vitamin D in the lab and add it to the milk.

4. The discontinuation of the treatment of milk with ultraviolet light appears to coincide with the start of an upward climb in the incidence of prostate and breast cancer.

INSULIN-
LIKE GROWTH
FACTOR ONE

I mentioned in the previous chapter that IGF-1 may be the major killer with estrogens as the accomplice. In fact, there have been no studies that link increased blood-serum levels of estrogens to prostate cancer. A Dutch-Japanese case-control study found that although estrogen levels were higher in the Dutch men studied, there were no differences between estrogen levels in the Dutch men with prostate cancer and those without the cancer. A similar finding occurs when the Japanese men with prostate cancer are compared to those without prostate cancer. These findings would seem confusing if estrogen was the main biochemical behind the development of prostate cancer and breast cancer. We must look more deeply into the deadly mix of proteins and hormones that exist in milk and other dairy products. It is the combination of IGF-1 and estrogens that gives us the breast, prostate, and other cancers. I will prove this to you with my presentation of what is already known. This is about science! *This is about peer-reviewed science.* This means other scientists who understand what is being said in the papers cited believe that the information you are about to read is correct.

Remember Grosvenor's work cited earlier? He and his fellow authors listed insulin-like growth factor-1 as one of the other agents in cow's milk.[2] *With this in mind, IGF-1 levels have been linked to an increased risk of prostate cancer.*

In the article by Shaneyfelt and other researchers, it is stated that "epidemiologic studies unequivocally link serum insulin-like growth factor-1 (IGF-1) levels with risk for prostate cancer."[3] A similar correlation was found among premenopausal women with breast cancer.[4] Stop to think about what has just been said by serious scientific research! The material knocked out by ultraviolet light (IGF-1) has been linked to breast and prostate cancer. Let us now take a look at this potent killer or, as I believe, the trigger-pulling protein that starts the cancer developing process.

Insulin like growth factor one (IGF-1) is a protein with hormone-like properties. It is folded on itself like a coiled snake and is held in this configuration by three sulfur-sulfur links (disulfide bonds), as previously described. It gets its name from the structural resemblance to insulin. It is mainly produced in the liver but also exists naturally in human breast milk.

IGF-1 levels vary widely in the bloodstream and are influenced by exercise, diet, and age. It is a potent stimulator of cells dividing, and the highest levels exist during teenage years. The levels drop off in older age.[5] IGF-1, which is secreted in human milk, is identical to that secreted in cow's milk and consists of exactly the same seventy-amino acid sequence. This protein hormone is very heat stable and is not destroyed during pasteurization.[6] This is an important point. Significant heat does not destroy IGF-1.

IGF-1 is carried in the bloodstream attached to one of six different binding proteins. They are labeled one through six, with insulin like growth factor binding protein three being the most common. Approximately eighty-five percent of IGF-1 in the bloodstream is bound to binding protein three. The function of IGF-1 depends on which binding protein it is attached to. Binding protein three is also found in human milk and as fragments in seminal fluid (more on this later).[7] It is generally the free-circulating IGF-1 that causes the actions associated with this protein hormone. Obviously then, the more free-circulating IGF-1, the greater the end effect. Again, I want to emphasize that when IGF-1 is not attached to a binding protein, it is free to wreak havoc. That havoc can involve starting the development of breast and prostate cancer.

As mentioned earlier, numerous studies have associated elevated serum levels of IGF-1 with prostate cancer. A study by Chan published in 1998 followed 152 cases (men with cancer) and 152 controls (men without cancer) in which blood was collected prior to the study. These men were watched for the development of prostate cancer. The blood collected prior to the study was then assayed for the levels of IGF-1. The study revealed that the men in the highest one-fourth of levels of IGF-1 had 4.3 times the risk of developing prostate cancer as men with levels of IGF-1 in the lowest one-fourth.[8] If you have more IGF-1 in your blood, then you have a higher risk of getting prostate cancer. Remember you have a lot of IGF-1 in dairy.

Shaneyfelt analyzed all published studies where men were age matched and other hormonal factors were adjusted, according to body weight, and concluded that men in the upper one-fourth of serum IGF-1 levels were at a twofold greater risk of developing prostate cancer.[9]

Acromegaly is a disease caused by a tumor in the pituitary gland in which increased levels of IGF-1 are released into the bloodstream. Jenkins states in a 2006 journal article that "There is some evidence to suggest that breast and prostatic malignancies might also be increased in acromegaly."[10]

There are also diseases in which occur congenital deficiencies of IGF-1. In a paper by Shevah et al. published in 2006, a review of the medical history of such patients revealed that none had malignancies. Further review revealed that 9–24 percent of family members without the deficiency had cancer. The conclusion of the paper was that "Congenital IGF-1 deficiency acts as a protecting factor for the development of cancer."[11] In other words, if you have a genetic defect where you cannot make IGF-1, you are not likely to get cancer.

Signorello and other researchers, in a 2000 review, linked height with an increased risk for prostate cancer

ROBERT BIBB, MD

in elderly men. These authors stated that: "The positive association between IGF-1 and height integrates the empirical evidence linking IGF-1 and height with prostate cancer risk."[12] IGF-1, of course, is also responsible for bone growth and, therefore, height. In other words, if you are taller, you probably have more IGF-1 and might be at higher risk for prostate cancer. I guess if you are a retired tall basketball player you might want to see your doctor.

In an interesting study reported by Majeed et al. in 2005, a group of mice was bred to be genetically predisposed to prostate cancer, and then a genetic impairment of the ability of IGF-1 to bind its receptors in prostate tissue was developed. There was a significant decrease in the percentage of mice showing changes for early cancer at thirty-five weeks of age.[13] In summary, if IGF-1 cannot attach to its receptors on your prostate or breast cells, it is less likely to cause cancer.

Finally, from a country other than the U.S, noted for its high incidence of prostate cancer and high per-person consumption of dairy, we find an interesting study. Stattin from Sweden, in a review in which blood was drawn from men without prostate cancer and then they were followed for an average of five years before prostate cancer developed, found that for men younger than 59 at time of blood drawing there was a 4.12 greater likelihood of developing prostate cancer if the IGF-1 level was in the upper one-quarter compared to the lower one-quarter.[14] *That is, a higher IGF-1 at a younger age predicts a greater risk of prostate cancer.*

I think it can be reasonably concluded that the blood levels of this IGF-1 protein are strongly related to the development of prostate cancer and that the levels of IGF-1 contained in the bloodstream of a man are proportional to his risk of developing prostate cancer.

Parents must be aware that by feeding their sons and daughters dairy products that they are feeding them a harmful mix of hormones and hormone-like proteins (IGF-1) in their diet. The question remains: are your children absorbing IGF-1 from their macaroni and cheese, milkshakes, yogurt, pizza, body-building protein shakes, and cheeseburgers? Let us take a look at the evidence to convince you that they are.

I will start with animal models first and then correlate these studies from what we know in humans. In one of the first animal studies, Xu looked at the oral-gastric (via a tube) administration of human IGF-1 to newborn and three-day-old piglets. This human IGF-1 was tagged with radioactive iodine so that the radioactivity could be traced. These authors found that a significant portion of the radioactive IGF-1 was found in the plasma (liquid portion) of the bloodstream, and most was bound to binding proteins. This indicated to the authors that IGF-1 can be absorbed through the gut of these piglets.[15] I will point out that pigs and humans behave very similarly as far as their biologic makeup. So if baby pigs can absorb IGF-1, so can human babies. So despite claims to the contrary, it is very likely that humans are absorbing IGF-1 from the dairy in their diet. The more dairy you eat, the more IGF-1 you absorb and the greater your risk of cancer.

In an interesting study by Philipps in 1997, the author administered rat pups either a rat milk substitute that contained no growth factors or the same milk substitute with human IGF-1 added and found that the serum concentrations of IGF-1 in the IGF-1 supplemented group were twice that of the rat milk substitute group with no IGF-1 added.[16] This would appear to imply that IGF-1 is absorbed because if it were not absorbed, then the IGF-1 levels in both groups should be the same.

In another rat study by Kimura in 1997, the authors looked at the absorption of radioactive human IGF-1 in these animals after oral feeding and found that there was a significant absorption of the radioactive IGF-1 into the blood of the rats. Additionally, the coadministration of casein enhanced significantly the absorption of the human IGF-1.[17] Casein is a mixture of compounds in the fat-soluble protein portion of milk and apparently enhances the absorption of its sister protein: IGF-1.

In 2000 Philipps studied the absorption of human radioactive IGF-1 in rats by measuring radioactive levels of the IGF-1 in the large artery entering the liver after the blood had drained into it from the intestinal tract. These authors concluded that, "It is likely that at least milk-borne IGF-1 is absorbed intact."[18] What can I say? Another animal study supports the absorption of human IGF-1 unchanged directly into the bloodstream.

Enough of the animals, you say! Well, now let us take a look at what we know about humans, dairy consumption, and IGF-1 levels.

The information we have on dairy consumption and IGF-1 levels comes mostly from incidental studies, looking at the impact of dairy on other tissues. There is one important study where the authors looked specifically at IGF-1 and other factors absorbed from dairy. I will detail this last, as I consider this the final piece of convincing evidence that humans are absorbing IGF-1 intact from their dairy intake.

First, Codogan and colleagues looked at milk supplementation on bone mineral density in eighty-two teenage women. These young women were divided into two groups. Both groups had been consuming an average daily milk intake of 150 milliliters (5 ounces). The first group continued to consume 150 milliliters of milk per day while the second group was given, on average, an additional 300 milliliters of milk (total of 15 ounces). They were followed over an eighteen-month period. Factors that were measured included blood levels of IGF-1. The levels of IGF-1 increased by 10 percent in the girls consuming 15 ounces compared to 5 ounces.[19] Two glasses of milk in the U.S. is 14 ounces. This should make milk-pushing parents uncomfortable. Remember that IGF-1 behaves like a hormone and that a 10% increase in IGF-1 in the blood could behave like the bowling ball effect described earlier.

In a study by Heaney and fellow researchers in 1999, the authors looked at 204 healthy men and women ages fifty-five to eighty-five who consumed on average one and a half servings of dairy foods per day. These people were asked to increase their consumption to three servings per day of nonfat or one percent milk over a twelve-week period. The blood levels of specific factors were measured during the course of the observation period. Of course, IGF-1 levels were measured, and when baseline levels were compared to increased milk consumption levels, a 10 percent increase in IGF-1 was noted.[20] It doesn't seem to matter whether you are young, old, male, or female: you are going to increase your IGF-1 levels by milk and other dairy consumption.

The final piece of information that I will present is a study by Rich Edwards and other researchers in which ten- to- eleven-year-old school girls in Mongolia and six- to eight-year-old school girls in Boston had blood levels of IGF-1 measured before and after milk consumption. Mongolian girls were assayed after one month of drinking 710 milliliters (about three glasses) daily of whole milk and in the Bostonian girls after drinking 710 milliliters of 2 percent milk compared to drinking a milk substitute for one week. The Mongolian girls had a mean increase in IGF-1 of 23.2 percent and the Bostonian girls of 5.2 percent.[21] The only conclusions one can draw from this study and the other papers outlined is that the average milk consumption increases plasma levels of IGF-1 by a minimal average of 10 percent and that the IGF-1 is absorbed into the bloodstream intact! IGF-1 is a powerful molecule, and a 10 percent increase does not result in a 10 percent increase in its effect. Through the secondary messenger system, as mentioned earlier, a many magnitude effect can occur.

We have now shown that serum IGF-1 levels parallel the incidence of prostate and premenopausal breast cancer and that dairy increases the levels of IGF-1 in serum. Let me show you now what this protein hormone does to your breast and prostate cells.

In our body there are genes that make things grow (oncogenes), and there are genes that make things die (suppressor genes). These genes can be turned on and off through chemical processes, as described earlier. This becomes a useful strategy for making a baby develop. It is the turn-off and turn-on of these genes that, for example, makes a hand appear with normal fingers. One of the major genes involved in making things grow and die is the so-called p53 gene. Not only does this gene help determine that we develop normally in the womb, but it later regulates normal cell division.

The p53 gene is an extremely important gene. This gene has been called the "guardian of the genome."[22] What is meant by this is that this gene, in particular, is very special in that one of the jobs it performs is to recognize when a cell becomes malignant. Once the p53 gene recognizes a malignant cell, it causes it to die by a method called *apoptosis*. Apoptosis causes cells to be reabsorbed with the contents being, in essence, reusable. This is a useful strategy for recycling cellular components without injuring healthy neighboring cells. This is the main strategy used to prevent cancer from developing. This type of death contrasts to necrosis, where the cellular contents are released by a literal explosion of a cell with injurious consequences to adjacent cells. The p53 gene should be thought of as the anticancer or major suppressor gene.

It would seem a reasonable thought that we want our p53 genes to be working well. One of the major influences on the p53 gene is through IGF-1, its binding proteins, and the receptor for the IGF-1 on our cells. Although on the surface, it may seem confusing that to allow a cell or group of cells to grow segments of the p53 gene must be inactivated or turned off. Are you confused yet? Remember the p53 gene in the on position causes cells to die. To allow cells to grow, you must turn the p53 gene off.

Remember, it is the free IGF-1 that exerts a powerful influence on cellular dynamics. This free IGF-1 does so by attaching to a receptor on breast or prostate cells. Adams points out that the binding of IGF-1 to its receptor protects cells from apoptosis (death). If cells are forced to develop more receptors for IGF-1, then in tissue cultures the cells become malignant.[23]

I mentioned earlier that one of the primary events occurring at the cellular level in prostate cancer is silencing of segments of the p53 gene.[24] This is accomplished through chemical turn-off of the little switches called CpG islands. The article cited above also postulated that, if we decrease the number of IGF-1 receptors back to normal or perhaps decrease the levels of IGF-1, we might be able allow the cancerous cells to die via apoptosis (programmed cell death).[25] This is a very important concept because I believe that this exactly is what happens when we intervene by treating prostate cancer patients with the dietary interventions. I will discuss these interventions later.

The importance of the p53 gene cannot emphasized enough. The p53 gene and its association with IGF-1, the IGF-1 binding protein, and the cellular receptors that receive IGF-1(IGF-IR) are intimately associated with the development of prostate cancer.[26] Mendouncesa-Rodriquez and fellow researchers point out that the absence of or mutations in the P53 gene result in increased tumor formation and further point out that 50–55 percent of all types of human cancer have defects in the p53 gene.[27] As confirmed previously, these p53 defects occur in prostate cancer.[28] The same defects have been reported in breast cancer.[29]

Other authors have looked at what happens when you inhibit the number of IGF-1 receptors in prostate cancer tissue and have found that you increase the IGF-1-binding protein.[30] Remember that if you increase the binding proteins for IGF-1, then you decrease free IGF-1. It is the free IGF-1 that wreaks havoc.

A normally functioning p53 gene is also capable of stimulating formation of the IGF-1-binding protein-3, which then binds the IGF-1. This process then prevents free IGF-1 from stimulating cells to become cancerous.[31]

I will repeat the mantra: free IGF-1 wreaks havoc.

It would also appear then that the IGF-1 receptor development on cells is an extremely important part of the picture in developing prostate cancer, breast cancer, and other cancers as well. Remember that Adams and others found that increasing the number of the IGF-1 receptors in cultured prostate cells resulted in malignant transformation of these cells.[32]

Another mantra: if you have an increase in the number of IGF-1 receptors on your prostate cells, then more IGF-1 can attach to them. This increases your risk of prostate cancer.

We know that milk and milk products contain a lot of IGF-1.[33] We also know that IGF-1 does not increase the number of IGF-1 receptors.[34] What could create an increased amount of these receptors? If you guessed estrogens, you would be right! Let us look at the evidence. And let me reinforce the concept that if you have more receptors for IGF-1, then you have a greater chance of cancerous transformation of your cells.

Pandini and others in a 2007 article, found that the

ROBERT BIBB, MD

most powerful estrogen, 17 beta estradiol, was able to markedly increase the number of IGF-1 receptors in cultured prostate cancer cell lines and that this occurred via the stimulation of the alpha estrogen receptors.[35] Remember that 17 beta estradiol is available in milk in small amounts, but the abundant estrogen in milk (estrone sulfate) can be converted in the body to 17 beta estradiol. Also it is important to know that there are two different receptors for estrogens on cells that have these receptors. They are known as the alpha and beta estrogen receptors.

Surmacz and fellow researchers have confirmed in breast cancer that estrogen receptor alpha stimulation increases the number of IGF-1 receptors and that insulin-like growth factor-1 receptor stimulation by IGF-1 stimulates an increase in the number of estrogen receptor alpha receptors.[36] Since prostate and estrogen receptor-positive breast cancer tissue behave similarly in the laboratory, it is very likely that what is said about one is true of the other.

So now I have described a cross talk phenomenon for you in which estrogen increases the number of IGF-1 receptors and 17 beta estradiol increases the number of IGF-1 receptors through stimulation of the alpha estrogen receptor. Stimulation of the alpha estrogen receptor then increases the number of IGF-1 receptors. It sounds like a dog chasing its tail but with deadly consequences. Remember that milk and milk products contain both IGF-1 and estrogens. The dog chasing its tail likely results in breast and prostate cancer. These events are summarized in Table One.

Table One: IGF-1 and estrogen interactions after ingestion of dairy products

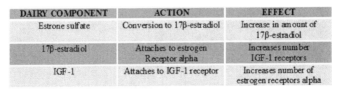

DAIRY COMPONENT	ACTION	EFFECT
Estrone sulfate	Conversion to 17β-estradiol	Increase in amount of 17β-estradiol
17β-estradiol	Attaches to estrogen Receptor alpha	Increases number IGF-1 receptors
IGF-1	Attaches to IGF-1 receptor	Increases number of estrogen receptors alpha

If the news about dairy described above is not bad enough, let me add one final piece of disturbing information about IGF-1 and gene activation. As there are genes that cause cancer cells to die, there are genes that can allow cancer cells to become immortal. These immortalizing genes are known as *oncogenes*. When you have a collection of cells that have become immortal (they do not die), then you have yourself a cancer. One of the most important oncogenes is called *bcl*-2. I described it earlier. It is called the bcl-2 gene because it was first described in B-cell leukemia/lymphoma. Every person is born with this gene, and if its presence in a cell is increased beyond normal, an increased risk for cancer will occur.

What could possibly increase the overabundance of bcl-2?

Yes, you guessed it! IGF-1 can increase bcl-2, or as we say in our technical papers, upregulate the expression of the bcl-2 gene. In fact, DiPaola and fellow scientists found that inactivation of the p53 can also lead to increased amounts of bcl-2 with a result that prostate cancer can become resistant to both chemotherapy and hormonal intervention. The inactivation of p53 and increased bcl-2 is seen more often in metastatic prostate cancer.[37] IGF-1 is indeed a potent protein that is involved in the cancer development process.

I have described, herein, the critical series of events mediated through the hormonal and protein factors in milk, which are believed to result in both prostate and breast cancer. There are certainly a cast of other supporting players consisting of both hormones and proteins that are believed to play a role in allowing hormonally sensitive cancer to develop. I believe that IGF-1 is the main killer, but it needs an accomplice. This would be estrogen.

What You Should Have Learned From This Chapter:

1. Serum IGF-1 levels correlate with prostate and premenopausal breast cancer incidence.

2. IGF-1 exists in significant levels in cow's milk and milk products.

3. IGF-1 is likely absorbed intact into the bloodstream from cow's milk.

4. IGF-1 and estrogens in cow's milk cause a reciprocal increase in the receptors for IGF-1 and estrogen receptor alpha.

5. IGF-1 causes the p53 gene, which is protective against cancer, to be inactivated. If you lose the effect of this gene, your cancer risk rises dramatically.

6. IGF-1 promotes the shutdown of the protective p53 gene. IGF-1 turns on the cancer causing gene bcl 2. Both of these events

increase the risk of prostate cancer and induce chemotherapy and hormone resistance to prostate cancer. This makes it very difficult to cure or stop your cancer from growing.

7. The stimulation of unbalanced numbers of estrogen receptors alpha by estrogens results in prostate cancer development. IGF-1 causes the increase in the number of estrogen alpha receptors. As an example, when a woman is said to have estrogen receptor positive breast cancer, what is being said is that she has too many alpha estrogen receptors. The increased number of the alpha receptors along with their stimulation by estrogens increases the growth of the cancer. For this reason Tamoxifen® is used to help block the receptors and increase survival in breast cancer.

ESTROGENS

Before I start this chapter I need to give the reader a primer on the terms used to describe the amounts of hormones in dairy:

A Short Primer on the Metric System:

Pico: One-trillionth

Nano: One-billionth

Micro: One-millionth

Milli: One-thousandth

Estrogens, being the predominantly female hormones, are generally thought of as being exclusively related to female fertility and as a component of birth control pills. This is a misconception. It is known that men also make estrogens and that the levels of estrogen(s) increase as a man ages. Prostate cancer most often occurs in older men, when the levels of estrogen(s) are at their highest. It has been presumed that these higher levels of estrogen are the result of the natural aging process and that prostate cancer is inevitable as a man reaches older age. I have even heard the statement that if a man lives long enough, he will eventually get prostate cancer. I will dispel that myth in this chapter and will summarize the current peer-reviewed research that nullifies the belief that male hormones cause prostate cancer. I will provide detailed information that it is the female counterpart (estrogens) consumed exogenously in concert with the other dairy proteins IGF-1 and likely PSA (prostate-specific antigen) that cause this disease. In a recent unpublished study, Dr. Lyndom Larcom at Clemson University found that the addition of 17 beta estradiol to prostate cancer tissue cultures significantly increased the growth rate of the cancerous cells. This experiment is something that strikes to the core of prostate and breast cancer development and growth. As I and others have said, it is the effect of estrogens along with IGF-1 that cause prostate and breast cancer.

There are three naturally occurring estrogens. They are estratriol, estradiol, and estrone. All have basic structures related to cholesterol and are generically known as sex steroids. Their basic chemical structures are diagramed below.[2]

Figure One: Estratriol.[3]

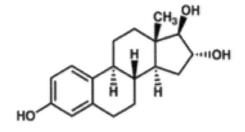

Figure Two: Estradiol.[4]

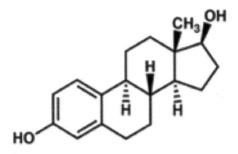

Figure Three: Estrone.[5]

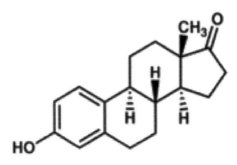

In women the most potent form of estrogen is *estradiol*. The most common form of estradiol is known as 17 beta estradiol. It can be created from testosterone through the action of an enzyme known as aromatase.[6] Estrogens are broken down in the bodies of mammals through metabolic processes that are mediated through certain enzymes. Through the action of these enzymes, both "good" and "bad" estrogen breakdown products can be created. The action of estrogen in women leads to the development of secondary sex characteristics, such as breast development, height, menstrual initiation, and bone formation. In a woman who has developed estrogen-sensitive breast cancer, estrogens can support its growth.[7] Remember that estrogen sensitive breast cancer means too many alpha receptors for estrogens.

To see the obvious effect of dairy-consumed estrogens on Western societies, just look at teenage women. They all look like they are eighteen or twenty in the seventh and eighth grades. The average age at which a U.S. woman starts her period is approximately 12.5 years.[8] If you compare the physical maturity of girls in the seventh grade to that of boys, there is a remarkable difference. My daughter lived in China and can testify that dairy products are an uncommon part of the Chinese diet. The average age at which a girl starts her period in rural China is around sixteen years of age.[9] If you think about it, estrogens are responsible for secondary sex characteristics in girls but not boys. Early puberty is occurring in girls in the U.S. I strongly believe this early puberty is because of the effects of estrogens in our dairy diets.

As I will explain in this chapter, estrogens are also intimately involved in the development of prostate cancer and are a normal component of the male hormonal system. Estrogens naturally increase in the bloodstream of a man as he ages. They are generated both endogenously (by our bodies naturally) and are also consumed exogenously (from the outside) through the ingestion of dairy products and beef.[10] Estrogens survive pasteurization.[11] These powerful hormones are contained in milk, the curds (casein) used in making cheese, whey (the liquid portion of milk), and butter.[12]

In a study done in the Netherlands, the total daily intake of estrogens from milk alone was estimated at 372 nanograms.[13] A nanogram is a billionth of a gram. Significantly higher intakes would occur when cheese, butter, and whey-containing products are consumed. In the Netherlands' study cited above, the method used to determine estrogen levels employed the modern method of extracting the estrogens and then using liquid chromatography in tandem with mass spectrometry (sounds complicated but highly accurate).[14] The levels of estrogens measured by this method are approximately tenfold greater than those measured in dairy products reported by Wolford and other scientists in 1979.[15] Daxenberger and fellow researchers reported on the estrogen levels in beef in a paper entitled "Possible Health Impact of Animal Estrogens In Food" in 2001, in which the most powerful estrogen 17 beta estradiol's theoretical maximum intake could reach 4.3 nanograms daily from nonestrogen-treated cattle.[16] This is a drop in the bucket compared to other levels of estrogens about to be discussed. This paper goes on to conclude that as much as twenty nanograms per day of this potent hormone could be consumed from beef-cattle treated with estrogens.[17] Treatment of cattle with estrogens is a common "good-animal-husbandry" practice used in the U.S.[18] Daxenberger's paper did not include all the other estrogens, such as estrone and 17 alpha estradiol, which have important health impacts.[19]

In a 2004 report, García-Peláez and fellow researchers reported on the total estrone content in dairy products and included the fat-soluble conjugated (conjugated means bound to something) estrogen in milk known as *oleoyl-estrone*. The levels of total estrone reported in the *Journal of Dairy Science* were high, and the concerned scientists ended their paper with the following quote: "The growth-inducing effects of milk-based diets for children may well be a consequence of its high-estrogen content."[20] In an animal study reported in 2008, Serrano-Muñounces and fellow researchers reported that oleoyl-estrone is well absorbed from the intestinal tract of rats.[21] Cabot and colleagues reported in 2007 that the main breakdown product of oleoyl-estrone in the body is estrone-sulfate.[22] Estrone sulfate is a water-soluble estrogen and would be found in high levels in skim or low-fat milk. It is a dangerous estrogen because enzymes in the body can convert into something more sinister.

In fact, if we look at how the prostate gland handles ingested and naturally existing hormones, it can be appreciated that estrone and testosterone can both be converted into 17 beta estradiol, the most potent natural estrogen. Estradiol and estrone can be converted from one to the other inside our body.

Figure Four: Conversion of estrone and testosterone to

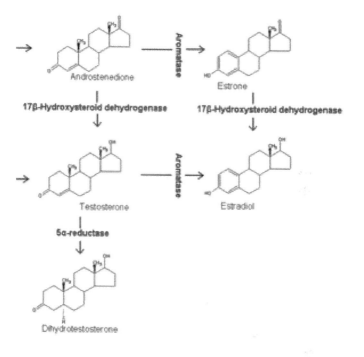

17 beta estradiol as occurs in the prostate gland.[23]

In the review of a paper by Henricks published in 1983, estrogen residues in beef cattle include estrone, 17 beta estradiol, and 17 alpha estradiol. [24] (Edible tissue would primarily include liver, fat, and muscle.) Henricks also points out that the concentrations of the estrogens vary according to the type of tissue studied and to the estrous cycle (equivalent to a women's menstrual cycle) and pregnancy phase of female cows (heifers). The levels of estrogens reported in this paper are higher in all tissues examined in steers injected with supplemental estrogens.[25] A summary of the estrogen concentrations in noninjected steers and heifers are listed in Table One. Since the conjugated and fat-soluble estrogen, oleoyl-estrone, had not been discovered yet and no reported analysis of its level in beef tissue is available, it is likely that the cattle tissue levels of estrogen are much higher.

Table One[26]: Estrogen residues in beef expressed in picograms per gram of each tissue, by Henricks, 1983

TISSUE TYPE	ESTRONE	17β-ESTRADIOL
Muscle	70.28	13.2
Fat	709.5	30.4
Liver	75.4	25.1

Table One: Summarized from data: Henricks, DM. "Endogenous Estrogens in Bovine Tissues," J of Animal Science 45 (1977): 652–8.[27]

The 17 beta estradiol levels reported in beef muscle by Hoffman and Karg (1976) in untreated calves was 100 picograms per gram, and in the liver assay the reported 17 beta estradiol level was 70 picograms per gram.[28]

In a study by Dunn and other scientists in 1977, cows were given radioactive estrogens, and the levels of radioactive estrogens were compared to raw beef after cooking. The residual levels of radioactive 17 beta estradiol were studied in raw, stewed, and roasted beef muscle. The residual radioactivity remained the same in all the specimens studied and extracted for this estrogen.[29] This would suggest that estrogen levels in cooked beef remain unchanged from those of raw beef, or more importantly, *estrogens may not be destroyed by cooking*. It has also been shown that estrogens are well absorbed through oral ingestion through the human gut.[30]

From the available knowledge of estrogen levels in beef tissue, a theoretical daily intake of total estrogen and possible absorption into the bloodstream of humans can be determined.

From USDA data, we know that the average beef consumption per capita per year is 63 pounds per year, or 78.4 grams per day. The average (low side) percentage of the beef that is fat is 11 percent. This would mean that our average daily meat consumption of 78.4 grams per day would have 8.6 grams of fat and 69.8 grams of muscle. Additional USDA data reveals that the per-capita (pounds per person), per-year consumption of additional tallow (melted fat) and beef fat is 5 pounds, or 6.2 grams per day.[31] This additional fat intake brings the total fat to 14.8 grams per day. Using the values for fat and muscle for estrogen levels by Henricks, the total daily intake of estrogens from beef alone equals 16.7 nanograms.[32] (See Appendix B.) Of course, the 16.7 nanograms number generated is just from the estrogens consumed from eating the cow's meat. We must now look at what cows deliver to us through ingestion of their milk and milk products. It becomes obvious that to avoid the harmful effects of dairy, beef must also be avoided.

There have been a number of studies that investigated the concentration of estrogenic steroids in consumable dairy products derived from milk and milk products. None of these studies looked at all of the estrogenic compounds in milk and milk-derived products, such as cheese, yogurt, etc.; however, this is the best data we have. I will summarize this data below and from this data will calculate a likely very conservative estimate on average daily intake of estrogen from milk and milk-derived products. Although beef contributes to the levels of hormones of concern, these levels are low compared to dairy products. I will give two calculations. One will include the information regarding the levels of estrone and estradiol estrogen levels. The second calculation will include values for oleoyl-estrone levels reported in the paper by García-Peláez.[33]

Table Two: Type of estrogen found in milk and author. Values are in picograms per milliliter

Estrogen and Source	Malekinejad 1	Wolford 2	Farlow 3	Narenden 4	Pape-Zambito 5	Daxenberger 6	Henderson 7
Estrone (E1)	6.2-1266	34-55	65.0-87.9	N/A	N/A	N/A	59
17α-Estradiol (E2)	7.2-322	N/A		N/A	N/A	N/A	N/A
17β-Estradiol (E2)	5.6-51	4-14	20.3-25.3	336-521	1.4	6.4	N/A

Sources: 1. Malekinejad H. et al., "Naturally occurring estrogens in processed and raw milk (from gestated cows)," Journal Agric Food Chemistry 54 (2006):9785–91. 2. Wolford ST. et al. "Measurement of estrogens in cow's milk, human milk and dairy products," Journal of Dairy Science 62 (1979):1458–63. 3. Farlow D. et al., "Quantitative Measurement of Endogenous Estrogen Metabolites, Risk-factors of development of Breast Cancer, in Commercial Milk Products," J of Chromatography B Analyt Technol Boimed Life Sci. 837 (2009):1327–34. 4. Narenden R. et al. "Hormonal induction of lactation: estrogen and progesterone in milk," Journal of Dairy Science 62 (1979): 1069–75. 5. Pape-Zambito DA. et al., "Concentrations of 17 -estradiol in Holstein whole milk," Journal of Dairy Science. 90 (2007):3308–13. 6. Daxenberger A., "Possible health impact of animal oestrogens in food," Human Reproduction Update. 7 (2001):340–55. 7. Henderson KM. et al., "Concentrations of oestrone sulfate during pregnancy in milk from Jersey and Freisian cows differing in milk yields and composition," New Zealand Vet. Journal. 42 (1994):89–92.

The total amount of milk marketed in 2005 was 169 billion pounds, and since milk is perishable, a large percentage (62 percent) was converted into milk-derived products, such as butter, cheese, and other dairy-related products.[34]

One way to look at the potential consumption per person would be to look at the total pounds of milk marketed and develop a per-capita consumption number based on that value. The per-capita consumption of each dairy product could also be used, but this would vastly underestimate the value because all of the numbers for per-capita consumption of all the products containing milk and milk-derived products are simply not available. Of course, not all marketed products are consumed. If I assume a conservative estimate that 50 percent marketed products are consumed, then let us take a look at what amount of estrogen on a daily basis might potentially enter our bloodstream.

What I have done in these calculations was to take the average value for each estrogen concentration developed from Table Two. Where an author has given us a range of values, I averaged that range first and then used that average combined with other single values to develop an overall average for the single estrogen compound. I then totaled all the estrogens as picograms (one-trillionth of a gram) per milliliter. So now let us take a look at the number we are after.

There are 8.6 pounds per gallon of milk. This gives us 19.65 billion gallons of milk marked per year (based on the marketed amount of milk in 2005).[35] The U.S. population was estimated at 293 million in 2005.[36] This would make the per person consumption of all dairy products at 67 gallons per year, or .18 gallons per day, per person, or 691 milliliters per person, per day. *With the average number of estrogens estimated at 428 picograms-per-milliliter in milk, then the total amount of estrogen consumed per day, per person in the U.S. is .31 micrograms.* If it is assumed that 50 percent of what is marketed is consumed, then this is still 0.16 micrograms per person, per day. This number may be on the low side considering that two 14-ounce glasses of milk per day (the size of a typical glass) equal 840 milliliters of this hormonal milieu per day. If we compare the 16.7 nanograms of estrogen consumed daily from beef, it becomes apparent that without considering oleoyl-estrone in beef tissue that dairy and dairy products are the major offenders.

Now let us take a look at the same calculation including the oleoyl-estrone. The average level of oleoyl-estrone when whole, lowfat, and skim milk are averaged is 403,000 picograms per mililiters.[37] This would give us 291 micrograms of estrogen per day in the average dairy diet! A low-estrogen birth control pill contains 35 micrograms of estrogen.

This is the equivalent of eight control pills' worth of estrogen! I certainly do not believe that all this estrogen is absorbed, nor do I believe that if it is absorbed it stays in an active form; but certainly some is metabolized into forms of estrogen that can be detrimentally contributing to an increased risk of prostate and breast cancer. (As an interesting side note, Ramesar and colleagues fed rats the equivalent of human oleoyl-estrone levels in a diet for fifteen days and found that the rats doubled their weight per day compared to rats not given this diet.)[38] Could it be that this weight-producing hormone in dairy is causing the obesity that we see in the U.S.?

Remember, I included the estimated entire U.S. population in my calculations. There are obviously much higher consumers of dairy, and there are also people who do not consume dairy. This would mean the actual average dairy consumption could be much higher. And lastly, parents are feeding their sons and daughters what could be on average perhaps 400 (assuming 50% marketing to consumption) percent of the estrogens in birth control pills without the knowledge that they are doing so. Realize that this number includes mostly the oleoyl-estrogens in one glass of 2% fat milk. Imagine what amount of estrogen could be consumed when eating pizza, milk on cereal, and a toasted cheese sandwich? In addition to adding to the eventual development of prostate and breast cancers in their sons and daughters, parents are causing premature development in their daughters, decreasing their daughter's fertility, and perhaps decreasing the fertility of their sons through a decrease in sperm counts. And just think about the potential problems with obesity that may occur as a result of dairy consumption. Parents are feeding themselves and their children levels of estrogens that perhaps exceed those in birth control pills by many times over.

In a peer-reviewed paper written by Pape-Zambito and fellow scientists in July 2007, the authors concluded that the levels of 17 beta estradiol in whole milk were too low to pose a health risk. In that paper, total estrogen levels were not assayed.[39] The conclusion by these authors may not be the general consensus among the scientific community. Daxenberger and his fellow researchers published a paper in 2001 expressing their concern about estrogens in food and estrogen as it relates to non-reproductive (such as cancer) functions.[40] In a an exhaustive review of the existing literature regarding dairy consumption and estrogen exposure in 2004, Li-Quang and fellow collaborators have provided significant evidence that estrogen exposure through dairy is related to prostate cancer development.[41]

The issue of whether the levels of estrogens in dairy are significant to have health impacts is being challenged almost daily by peer-reviewed research. In a recent article by Chavarro and cooperating scientists in 2007, it was revealed that in a prospective (examined as time went on) study of 18,555 enrolled women without infertility who were followed over an eight-year period that there was a significant percent increase in infertility associated with consumption of low-fat dairy products.[42] The obvious question that should be asked is: why would low-fat dairy be associated with decreased fertility? It becomes obvious when we look at how estrogens are secreted in milk.

Cows secrete estrogens in two forms. One form is as free, naturally occurring estrogens and their breakdown products and as other estrogens that are bound and are either fat soluble or water soluble. These would include oleoyl-estrone, which is a fat-soluble estrogen.[43] The others are also naturally occurring estrogens and their breakdown products, which are water soluble. An example of a water-soluble estrogen would include estrogen sulfate. These water-soluble estrogens are not removed during fat extraction from the milk. In a paper published in 2006 by Ganmaa and her fellow scientists it is pointed out that the main estrogen in milk is estrone sulfate, which is a water-soluble estrogen.[44] Other scientific studies have shown that estrone sulfate has a long half-life in the bloodstream of humans and, therefore, could prolong any estrogen effects.[45] The scientific paper by Ganmaa went on to show that in female rats commercial milk could affect the lining of the uterus.[46] Not only does milk have a suppressive effect on egg development (ovulation), thus behaving like a birth control pill, but it can affect the lining of the uterus, both of which would expect to decrease fertility. A Swedish cohort (remember more accurate than case-controlled) study found that women who consumed more than four servings of dairy per day doubled their risk of ovarian cancer.[47]

Remember at the beginning of this book, I made a point in the introduction to suggest that dairy should be implicated in cancer of the prostate, breast, uterus, testes, and ovaries. The process is likely carried out through estrogen receptors in these tissues in a process similar to that described by Ganmaa above.[48] Why am I talking about the lining of the uterus, ovarian cancer, and breast cancer in a book about prostate cancer? This is why: all the hormonally sensitive tissues, such as breast, edometrium (lining of the uterus), prostate, ovarian, and testicular, have estrogen receptors alpha that could react negatively to received estrogens. Certainly, prostate and estrogen receptor positive breast cancers behave in a similar fashion when exposed to estrogens, and that response is to cause abnormal cell division. In other words, cancer development.

For years, it has been assumed that prostate cancer was an androgen-mediated (male hormone) disease, but there is no consistent evidence that this is the case.

As Carruba points out in his article entitled "*Estrogen and Prostate Cancer: An Eclipsed Truth in an Androgen-Dominated Scenario*": "The association between plasma androgens and prostate cancer remains contradictory and mostly not compatible with the androgen (male hormone) hypothesis."[49]

The mechanisms regarding the negative impact that estrogens have on prostate tissue and the likely processes resulting in prostate cancer have been revealed in a number of scientific papers.

Risbridger and his fellow scientists eloquently describe the negative impact estrogens have on prostate tissue on multiple levels.[50] The estrogens are released by three different mechanisms I previously described. They include endocrine, paracrine, and autocrine processes. Endocrine implies that hormones such as estrogens are directly released into the bloodstream by certain signaling systems. These estrogens circulate throughout the body. They are released directly from our ovaries, testes, and adrenal glands. I would add that exogenous (from outside our body) estrogens are added to our bloodstream from ingestion of dairy and would essentially be indistinguishable from those naturally released.

Paracrine release (*para* meaning "next to") of estrogens occurs in the prostate stroma or connective tissue where an enzyme known as *aromatase* converts the male hormone testosterone to estrogen.

Autocrine refers to a dangerous process in which the cells of prostate cancer start making estrogen spontaneously without inhibition. The malignant cells comprising the prostate cancer are then essentially feeding themselves estrogen. Remember that Dr. Larcom showed in his experiment that estrogen significantly promoted the growth of prostate tissue.[51] Estrogens produced in the variety of mechanisms described, herein, will influence the prostate gland through recently characterized estrogen receptors. The receptors have been labeled as estrogen receptor alpha and estrogen receptor beta. Stimulation of each individual receptor can have vastly different impacts on prostate tissue. Most of the negative effects are mediated through stimulation of the alpha-estrogen receptor. These include increased cell division, such as prostate enlargement. An enlarged prostate is the reason for men having hesitancy and urinary frequency. Another negative stimulatory effect of estrogen receptor alpha is inflammation. This leads to prostatitis, which is inflammation of the prostate gland. Inflammation can promote prostate cancer development. Lastly, one of the main results of estrogen alpha receptor stimulation by estrogens is abnormal cell division of prostate cells that likely leads to prostate cancer. Stimulation of estrogen receptor beta, on the other hand, will have positive effects on the prostate gland, such as preventing enlargement, preventing inflammation, and likely helping prevent prostate cancer.[52]

As a side note, when a woman is said to have estrogen-receptor-positive breast cancer, it is implied that this means an excess number of estrogen receptors alpha.

You may be thinking: if we have equal numbers of alpha and beta receptors in the prostate gland, why wouldn't their effect be cancelled out by estrogen stimulation and the gland remain normal? That would be an excellent question. Estrogens are killers, but to accomplish their task, they need an accomplice. Remember

Grosvenor's work on dairy cited earlier? He analyzed milk for various hormones and proteins and listed insulin-like growth factor one as an ingredient.[53]

Estrogens certainly can be killers, but to accomplish their task they need additional assistance. I described previously how an increased imbalance in favor of increased alpha receptors occurs on prostate cells through exposure to insulin-like growth factor one. This imbalance results in increasing the risk for development of prostate cancer. The imbalance in estrogen receptor alpha that helps lead to prostate cancer is just part of the story. I now have to introduce to you the estrogen metabolites or breakdown products.

When mammals ingest materials that may be toxic to the body, there are enzyme systems designed to detoxify and eliminate these materials. The enzymes systems are grouped into two categories. They are called phase-one and phase-two systems. The basic job of phase one is to detoxify a chemical, and phase-two enzymes then prepare the chemical for elimination from the body through excretion through water-soluble pathways using the kidneys or fat-soluble pathways using the intestines. The name given to the chemicals created through these pathways is metabolites. Many of the chemicals broken down to metabolites include both endogenous (naturally occurring in our body) and exogenous (taken in through the diet) chemicals. The chemicals of interest for this discussion include estrogens and their metabolites generated both naturally within our body or consumed through dairy products.

A number of the phase-one and -two enzymes have been characterized, and their metabolites have been studied. I mentioned earlier that there are both "good" estrogens and "bad" estrogens. These are the metabolites of estrogens that will be discussed. These "good" and "bad" estrogens are characterized in terms of their beneficial or detrimental effects based on how they attach to the previously described alpha- or beta-estrogen receptors.

In his article *"Estrogen's Two-Way Street,"* Dan Lukaczer has characterized this process of estrogen metabolism.[54] The three naturally occurring estrogens estrone, estradiol, and estratriol can be considered as the parent compounds, and these can be broken down into good daughter compounds and bad daughter compounds by attaching an OH (hydroxyl group) to certain points in the estrogen molecules. As Dan Lukaczer writes,

> Estrogen molecules are composed of carbon ring structures that are named numerically. Estradiol has 17 carbon atoms and can be hydroxylated (OH group attachment) at particular points on that ring. Considerable research has shown that major metabolites of estradiol and estrone are those hydroxylated at either the C2 (carbon number 2 position) or the C16 (carbon number 16 position). Hydroxylated (OH group attached) metabolites at the C4 position are also present, but in lesser amounts. We might think of this process as parent estrogens (estradiol and estrone) begetting daughter estrogens C2, C4 and C16. The daughter compounds would then be referred to

as hydroxyestrones or hydroxyestradiols depending on the original parent estrogen. The problem is that some of these daughter estrogens are the "good" daughters and some are the "bad" daughters.[55]

The enzymes that are responsible for converting estrogens into the good C2 "daughter estrogens" are called *CYP1A*1 and *CYP1A*2. The enzymes that are responsible for converting estrogens into the C4 and C16 "bad daughter estrogens" are known as *CYP3A*4 and *CYP1B*1.[56]

A commercial urine test has been developed, which can measure the ratio of the C2 to C16 metabolites of estrone.[57] Since C2 is "good" as far as preventing cancer and C16 is "bad as far as stimulating cancer," it becomes obvious that the larger the ratio, the less likely a person is to get cancer. The amount of CYP enzymes 1A1 and 1A2 that create a favorable ratio can be increased by a process known as *induction*. Induction can occur through ingestion of dairy. Using dairy consumption would be a bad way to induce or increase the enzymes because "bad" estrogens will be created. A more favorable process of induction would include eating certain vegetables, such as broccoli or kudzu.[58] Yes, I did write the word *kudzu*. The vine that is considered a nuisance in the U.S. could save your life!

The "good" daughter and "bad" daughter effects of the metabolites of estrogens are created by the preferential stimulation of alpha and or beta estrogen receptors and have been characterized in a scientific article by Bao Ting Zhu and fellow researchers at the University of South Carolina.[59] I consider this a seminal article in explaining how dairy estrogens can injure humans by causing prostate and breast cancer. This article also explains how soy phyto-estrogens (plant based) may be beneficial.

There is a technique to look at estrogens as to whether one type of estrogen compound or metabolite is more or less "estrogenic" than another. One test can look at how well certain estrogen compounds stimulate breast cancer cells to grow. Using this test and comparing the natural estrogens, the lineup would be estratriol as least powerful, estrone as second most powerful, and estradiol as the most powerful.

Remember that it is the attachment of estrogens to the estrogen receptors alpha and beta that determines cell proliferation.[60] It is a generality that the *estrogenicty* (strength) of certain compounds is determined on how they bind to the estrogen receptor alpha.

These processes become very complex if we have something causing an imbalance of receptors. This attachment process becomes even more complex if a particular estrogen preferentially attaches to an alpha or beta estrogen receptor. Further complexity occurs when a particular estrogen attaches to a receptor and acts as a blocking agent so that cancer chances are reduced. I will try to clear up this confusing process by looking at what the peer-reviewed research has already demonstrated.

It is already known that estrogens and insulin-like growth factor one act in a reciprocal fashion to increase the number of estrogen receptors alpha on prostate cells (and likely breast cells). We also know that attachment of certain estrogens to estrogen receptor alpha results in prostate cells being stimulated to become abnormal or frankly malignant.[61] What we do not know is how certain estrogens, their metabolites (daughter estrogens) or plant-based estrogens bind to these receptors. Let us take a look at what Dr. Zhu and colleagues have found regarding the ability of these materials to bind to their receptors.[62]

I am going to look at naturally occurring estrone and 17 beta estradiol as well as their metabolites. I will also take a look at Tamoxifen®, which is used as an estrogen-blocking agent in estrogen receptor positive breast cancer. Genistein and daidzein are two plant-based estrogenic compounds found in soy. This is our list:

1. Estrone

2. 17 beta estradiol

3. 2-Hydroxyestrone (C2)– an estrone metabolite

4. 2-Hydroxyestradiol—an estradiol metabolite

5. 4-Hydroxyestrone—an estrone metabolite

6. 4-Hydroxyestradiol—an estradiol metabolite

7. 16 alpha Hydroxyestrone— an estrone metabolite

8. 16 alpha Hydroxyestradiol— an estradiol metabolite

9. Tamoxifen®

10. Daidzein

11. Genistein

I have adopted a modification of Dr. Zhu's measurements. Dr. Zhu and colleagues reported the binding capacity of estrogen metabolites differently than I am reporting them.[63] My reporting method is simply a way of comparing relative capacity of compounds to bind to estrogen receptors alpha and/or beta. I am using a scale of 1–200. The higher the number, the greater the affinity for a receptor. It becomes an easy exercise to determine which compound might have a negative impact on prostate tissue. If the binding affinity is greater for alpha, then a negative impact might be expected. If the binding is greater for beta, then a positive impact might be expected. There are exceptions in that that certain estrogens such as 2-hydroxestrone (C2), phytoestrogens (genistein and daidzein), or designed blocking agents such as Tamoxifen® that bind to alpha receptors are very weak estrogens and probably block the estrogen effect. Table Three lists the relative binding capacities.

Table Three: Relative binding capacities of estrogens and estrogen metabolites and other chemicals to estrogen receptors alpha and beta. Adapted from Zhu et al.[64]

Metabolite or Chemical	Relative α receptor binding capacity	Relative β receptor Binding capacity
estrone	11.2	44.7
17β-estradiol	1.1	0.89
2- Hydroxyestrone	31.6	199.5
2-Hydroxyestradiol	5.0	2.5
4-Hydroxyestrone	70.8	70.8
4-Hydroxyestradiol	1.6	1.6
16α-Hydroxyestrone	5.6	2.5
16α-Hydroxyestradiol	10	2.5
Tamoxifen	35.4	25.1
daidzein	100	63
genistein	19.9	1.1

Table Three: From a modification of Table 1 page 431 from Zhu and fellow researchers. "Quantitative Structure-Activity Relationship of Various Endogenous-Estrogen Metabolites for Human Estrogen Receptor, and Subtypes: Insights into the Structural Determinants Favoring a Differential Subtype Binding."

I am going to point out several things about Table Three. You must first remember that generally if we stimulate alpha receptors by an estrogen this is going to produce a situation that causes cancer. If we stimulate beta receptors by an estrogen, this is going to produce a situation that decreases the chance of cancer. If we look at the table, it becomes obvious that 2-hydoxyestone (C2) stimulates beta receptors to a much greater degree than alpha receptors. This favors a situation that decreases risk of cancer. This would be considered a "good" daughter. Now look at 16 alpha hydroxyestone (C16). The binding of C16 favors estrogen receptor alpha. This would be considered a "bad" daughter. Now you know why the C2 to C16 ratio is important, and we can measure it in the urine!

Now take a look at Tamoxifen®, daidzein, and genistein. They have binding affinities that favor estrogen receptor alpha. They should be bad. It turns out that these compounds do not behave as estrogens (not estrogenic) when they attach to estrogen receptor alpha. In fact, they block the effects of estrogens at the alpha-receptor site. That is why Tamoxifen® is used in estrogen receptor positive breast cancer.

I have written previously about how the body eliminates compounds by converting them through the phase-two enzyme pathway. This is also how mammals eventually eliminate estrogens. Let me go over this again. First the animal takes the natural estrogens estrone and 17 beta estradiol, converts them into "good" or "bad" estrogens, and then converts these to other compounds, which are eliminated from the body. These "final" estrogens are converted into what are known as *methoxyestrogens.*

Farlow and colleagues have reported on the "final" estrogen metabolites in cow's milk and found that the levels of these metabolites are high. They reported that the methoxyestrogens were extremely high.[65]

Methoyestrogens in milk can have a negative influence on the C2 to C16 ratio. Dawling and colleagues at Vanderbilt University reported on the feedback mechanisms of methoxyestrogens on our "favorite" enzyme, CYP1A1. Feedback is a term used to describe how a compound might turn a particular enzyme "off." These researchers found that as CYP1A1 converts estrogens to "good" estrogens, the next step, which is conversion to methoyestrogens, results in turn-off of CYP1A1.[66] This feedback process in this instance is dangerous. This is because it is turning "off" an enzyme that manufactures a "good" estrogen.

We now have another piece of the puzzle on how dairy may contribute to prostate cancer. The methoxyestrogens turn off CYP1A1, which now cannot convert estrogens to the "good" daughters. Navas and fellow colleagues also showed that 17 beta estradiol also turns off CYP1A1, resulting in decrease of the "good" daughter C2.[67] We already know that milk contains high levels of 17 beta estradiol.

Another enzyme known as *CYP1B1* can convert estrogens into the "bad" daughter, C16.[68] This CYP1B1 enzyme is stimulated to develop or be *induced* by the estrogen receptor alpha.[69] We have already seen how IGF-1 and estrogens cause an increase in estrogen receptor alpha.[70] It has been demonstrated that the zones of the prostate gland, which are cancerous, exhibit high levels of this CYP1B1 enzyme.[71] Remember that this enzyme manufactures the "bad" C16 estrogen. I would make the claim that prostate and breast-cancer likely occur through the breakdown of estrogens that are consumed in dairy products along with IGF-1 that is also contained in dairy products. The human body has not evolved to handle such enormous quantities of estrogens and IGF-1 consumed in dairy products. The body does what it knows how to do and that is to eliminate these estrogens. Unfortunately in the elimination process the balance of "good" to "bad" estrogens is greatly disturbed and prostate and breast cancer and likely other cancers such as ovarian and others result. In summary, I can say that insulin-like growth factor one in concert with estrogens likely cause these cancers. Dairy products have high levels of both.

As an additional note, the process I just described may account for the protective effects noted with dairy consumption and colon cancer. In the gut it has been theorized that CYP1A1 takes compounds in cooked animal proteins and converts them to more carcinogenic (dangerous) compounds. If dairy estrogen (methoxyestrogen) turns off CYP1A1, this would be a benefit in prevention of colon cancer. You would, however, be trading reduced risk of colon cancer for prostate, breast, and ovarian cancers. It would be like trading a risk of lung cancer for weight loss by smoking.

I have now taken you through the likely series of events and mechanisms on how estrogens, their breakdown products and insulin-like growth factor one are likely to be involved in the process of cancer development.

Let us now look at other likely supporting events.

☠

What You Should Have Learned From This Chapter:

1. Estrogens are naturally secreted by cows in their milk.

2. Estrogens can be water or fat soluble and can be in skim or fat-free dairy products.

3. Estrone and estradiol are interchangeable and that total estrogen content in dairy must be considered when looking at total estrogens consumed.

4. Estrogens are well absorbed from the human gut.

5. Estrogens survive cooking.

6. Estrogens can have beneficial or harmful effects on the prostate gland.

7. Estrogen receptor beta stimulation has a beneficial effect.

8. Estrogen receptor alpha stimulation has a negative effect.

9. Estrogens can be broken down into "good" (C2) and "bad" (C16) estrogens.

10. The enzyme CYP1A1 can break down estrogens into the "good" daughter.

11. Methoxyestrogens in milk can potentially turn off CYP1A1.

12. Estrogens can turn of CYP1A1, decreasing the production of "good" C2.

13. Estrogens can turn on the enzyme CYP1B1, increasing the production of "bad" C16.

14. Prostate cancer is in part caused by the enzyme CYP1B1 converting the high levels of estrone in milk to a "bad" estrogen.

PROSTATE-SPECIFIC ANTIGEN

Prostate-specific antigen (PSA) is a protein produced in the prostate tissue. It was so named because after its discovery it was thought to be made only by the prostate gland. It turns out that it is not specific to the prostate but has been found in tissue fluid from the breast. It has also been detected in tissues from the thyroid gland, trachea, salivary gland, parts of the small intestine, urethra, pancreas, and skin.[1]

PSA belongs to a category of compounds known as kallikreins. These compounds behave as enzymes and have specific enzymatic functions. Prostate-specific antigen is secreted in seminal fluid. One of the functions of PSA is to digest a protein known as *semenogelin*, which like a gelatin (for which it is named) keeps sperm immobile. Liquefaction of the semen allows sperm to become more mobile.[2]

PSA is found in the bloodstream, and the normal values for this enzyme have been established by surveying a large number of men without prostate cancer. It has become established that 99 percent of men have levels not exceeding four nanograms per milliliter of serum (4ng/mililiter), or when stating the PSA value, the ng/mililiter is assumed, and we might say to a patient: "Your PSA is less than four."[3]

PSA analysis has become a way of determining whether a person's physician should suspect a man of having prostate cancer. A man whose PSA exceeds four might be evaluated further for existence of cancer. The problem is that one man's PSA might be normal at 1 or less than 1 and another normal at 3.8. This is because there is a large variation in PSA values in a normal population of men without prostate cancer. It can become a dilemma if only absolute values are used to become suspicious about whether a man has prostate cancer. The use of absolute values, as the only parameter, may subject a man to further evaluation that may be unnecessary.

Another standard being used is the so-called PSA velocity, which is defined as how much a man's PSA changes during serial analyses over time. In his article entitled *"PSA Velocity: Important New Tool in Fight Against Prostate"*[4], William J. Catalona, MD, states, "Those with a .75 PSA increase within a year show a worrisome risk for prostate cancer. Those with a 2.0 increase within a year are more likely to have an aggressive cancer with a higher potential for death."[5]

Unfortunately, there is no perfect lab test or noninvasive method, including absolute PSA, PSA velocity, or digital rectal exam, to detect early prostate cancer. More specific markers in the bloodstream are being investigated and may become commonplace. At this point, the best advice is to have an exam at least yearly by your physician where he can coordinate a digital rectal exam with a PSA test and send you to a urologic physician for prostatic ultrasound (sound waves) studies and/or a prostate biopsy procedure.

This chapter was not meant as a treatise on how to understand PSA testing, but it was written to allow you to understand the more serious, albeit sinister, function of PSA. Remember when we talked about insulin-like growth factor? I stated that it is mostly bound together with the main binding protein called insulin-like growth factor binding protein three. When it is bound it does not do the dirty work described previously. The free, or unbound, IGF-1 is the protein hormone that regulates the number estrogen receptors alpha leading to the development of prostate cancer.

☠

I have some additional bad news for you: PSA splits IGF-1 away from its binding protein three by enzymatically digesting the binding protein three. Remember that PSA is an enzyme. It may make your sperm swim more freely, but it can—in effect—also increase the risk of developing prostate cancer by increasing your free IGF-1.

It was discovered that PSA naturally exists in human breast milk in 1995.[6] With a suspicion that PSA might also be in cow's milk, I had commercial milk tested and found that *PSA does exist in cow's milk*. The analyses were performed by a commercial PSA-testing machine. The values were low and might be higher when more sophisticated tests are performed.

Why then do you think PSA would be in the milk of mammals, such as humans and cows? For the reason described above: PSA raises free IGF-1, and free IGF-1 makes the baby animal grow more quickly! So now you have PSA made by the prostate cancer, and you are likely drinking PSA in your milk. This creates more free IGF-1, which may not only help initiate prostate cancer but make your existing cancer grow faster. It becomes the proverbial dog-chasing-its-tail situation with PSA increasing free IGF-1, it in turn increases prostate growth, and this creates more prostate tissue to produce more PSA, etc.

Now let us look at the peer-reviewed literature to support what I have written about these phenomena. Aksoy and fellow scientists looked at the PSA cleavage of insulinlike-growth-factor-three process in a 2004 article and went on to state[7]:

> Insulin-like growth factor binding protein-3(IGFBP-3) is the major carrier protein in serum for IGF-1, thus is an important functional modulator of it. On the other hand, one of the functions of prostate-specific antigen (PSA) is to cleave IGGBP-3. Epidemiological studies have shown that decreased levels of serum IGFBP are associated with increased PC (prostate cancer) risk.[8]

This paragraph is stating what I just finished writing, and that is binding proteins tie up the IGF-1, and when IGF-1 is free, the risk of prostate cancer increases.

Remember the mantra: free IGF-1 wreaks havoc.

Cohen and his collaborators in 1994 studied what happens to IGF-1 when its binding protein three is cleaved and found that[9]:

> PSA decreases the affinity of IGFBP-3 for IGF-1 and can potentiate IGF-1 action in the absence of inhibitory IGFBP-3. This may contribute to normal and malignant prostate growth.[10]

Here we see that same statement made by other scientists.

From the investigations of Cohen and others in 1992 looking at seminal fluid, it was speculated that: "PSA may serve to modulate IGF function within the reproductive system or in prostate cancer by altering IGF-IGFBP-3 interactions.[11] In other words, PSA is behaving like an enzyme and splitting IGF-1 away from the binding protein. It is creating free IGF-1. Free IGF-1 is the "Grim Reaper."

And finally, Réhault and his scientists summarized the effect of PSA very well in a 2001 article.[12] They state:

> Insulin-like growth factors (IGFs) are important growth regulators of both normal and malignant prostate cells. Their action is regulated by six insulin-like growth factor binding proteins (IGFBPs). The proteolytic (enzymatic) cleavage of IGFBPs by various proteases (PSA) dramatically increases

their affinity for their ligands (binding sites) and; therefore, enhances the bioavailability of IGFs.[13]

Basically PSA is now freeing IGF-1 so that it can start to increase the number of estrogen receptors alpha above normal. The cancer process begins!

Note: Proteolytic cleavage is synonymous with digestion: in this case the binding protein three is digested by PSA.

Table One: PSA effect on IGF-1 and end result

ENZYME	MOLECULE DIGESTED	END RESULT
PSA	IGF-1 binding protein three	Releases IGF-1 from it binding protein three, effectively increasing free IGF-1

We have now looked at insulin-like growth factor one, estrogens, and prostate-specific antigen. You are now aware that they are in the dairy foods that you are consuming. Further analysis of milk by more accurate methods should demonstrate the presence of significant amounts of PSA.

There is a large difference in the incidence of prostate cancer between African-American patients and Caucasian patients in all countries where Western diets are consumed.[14] Using what I have already told you and some additional information, read on, and let me explain to you why this is so.

What You Should Have Learned From This Chapter:

1. Prostate-specific antigen (PSA) is an enzyme made by prostate tissue and other tissues in the body, including breast tissue.

2. PSA probably exists in cow's milk.

3. PSA measurement can be used to suspect prostate cancer.

4. PSA digests or cleaves IGF-1 binding protein from IGF-1, raising free IGF-1 levels.

5. PSA is an adaptive enzyme to help mammals, such as humans and cows, grow more quickly.

6. Free IGF-1 causes an increased number of estrogen receptors alpha.

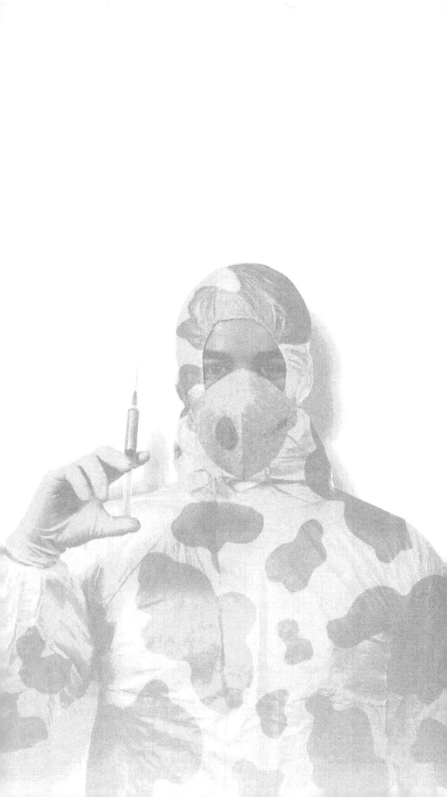

AFRICAN-AMERICAN MEN AND PROSTATE CANCER:

Multiple Jeopardies

The incidence of prostate cancer is significantly higher in African-American men than Caucasian men in the United States and is almost consistently approximately fifty percent higher for black men in any age group. This is graphically demonstrated in the U.S data graph below:

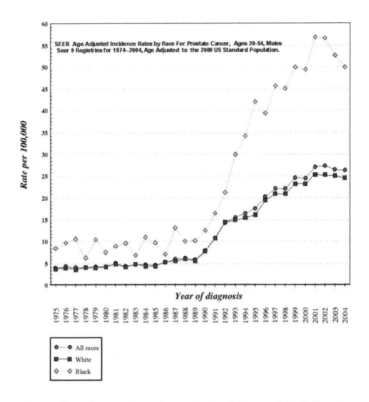

Figure One: Source: Surveillance, Epidemiology and End Results (SEER) Program U.S. Government. http://www.seer.cancer.gov.

African-English men in the United Kingdom also have a higher risk of prostate cancer than their Caucasian counterparts.[1] African-Caribbean men are three times more likely to be diagnosed with prostate cancer than their white counterparts.[2]

There is also a north-to-south gradient seen in the incidence of prostate cancer in both the African-American and Caucasian populations in the United States, with the highest levels found in the northern states. This is presented in Table One:

Table One: Prostate cancer incidence North-South Gradient Comparison Table

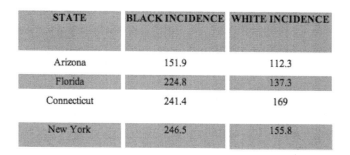

STATE	BLACK INCIDENCE	WHITE INCIDENCE
Arizona	151.9	112.3
Florida	224.8	137.3
Connecticut	241.4	169
New York	246.5	155.8

Source: http://statecancerprofiles.cancer.gov/
incidenceragtes/index.php?stateFIPS=36&cancer=066

Although data for African-American versus Caucasian incidence rates of prostate cancer for countries other than the U.S. are difficult to find, it can generally be appreciated that in any country looked at that African men will have significantly higher rates of prostate cancer than their Caucasian counterparts. It can also be appreciated that there is a trend toward lower rates of prostate cancer in warmer, albeit sunnier states. Why would African-American men have a higher incidence of prostate cancer in any given country, and why would they have higher rates in colder climates? Hint: It isn't the cooking!

Let me be serious, and let me take you through the science. As we discussed earlier, prostate cancer has been directly linked to higher levels of free IGF-1, the growth hormone. To get higher levels of free IGF-1, you could of course eat more food containing IGF-1. I think it would be foolish for me to suggest that African men in every country eat more dairy. Another way to get more free IGF-1 is to have less of the binding protein that ties up IGF-1. Remember that IGF-1-binding protein three is the major binding protein that ties up IGF-1? This is the first way in which black men are negatively impacted with higher prostate cancer rates because they are born with lower levels of this major binding protein three.

Winter and his scientists in 2001 looked at the levels of the IGF-1 binding protein three in African-American men, who were at increased risk of developing prostate cancer, and found these levels were low in this population at risk.[3] Statti and his collaborators in 2000 found that the higher the levels of IGF-1 binding protein three, the lower the risk of prostate cancer.[4] In 2007 Hernandez and his fellow researchers looked at the genes that influence the production of IGF-1 binding protein three in African-Americans and found that certain aspects of these genes resulted in lower levels of this important binding protein. They went on to further implicate lower IGF-1 binding protein three levels as playing a role in prostate cancer development.[5] In additional studies for IGF-1, Tricoli and scientists determined the IGF-1 binding protein three levels in age matched controls of Caucasian and African-American men and found that "IGF-1 binding protein-3 plasma levels are lower in African-American men than in Caucasian men."[6]

The first part of the triple jeopardy for development of prostate cancer in African-American men is their genetically lower levels of IGF-1 binding protein three. This is a genetically programmed deficiency. The second part of their jeopardy is that black men are born to be programmed to have higher levels of prostate-specific antigen (PSA).[7] Prostate-specific antigen is an enzyme, and, as stated earlier, it enzymatically digests or cleaves IGF-1 binding protein three away from IGF-1. This process effectively releases more free IGF-1. You will remember that free IGF-1 is the form that will cause a cascade of events resulting in prostate cancer. Let me summarize these concepts in the table below:

ETHNICITY	BIOLOGIC PROCESS	BIOLOGIC PROCESS	EFFECT
BLACK	↓ Binding Protein	↑PSA	↑Incidence of prostate cancer
CAUCASIAN	Normal binding protein	Normal PSA	Expected incidence of prostate cancer

And why would black men and women have higher levels of PSA and lower levels of binding protein three?

If, as a race, African men (and women) evolved as the first humans on the plains of Africa, it would make sense to have an evolutionary biological system that would allow a newborn human to develop maturity and survivability as quickly as possible. This system would be necessary because if animals larger than you were hunting you, faster maturation would increase survivability. Such a system would be designed to increase free IGF-1. This is exactly what we see in African-American men and women. This would be a great system to insure species survival under the pressure of predation (hunting you) but just might present a problem as history moved forward into a dairy-consuming population. The problem of greatly increased rates of prostate cancer is exactly what has happened to Africans migrating from Africa to the United States. As Oedina and other researchers point out in their 2006 article, compared to Nigerian men, African-American men have a greater than tenfold greater risk of developing prostate cancer.[8] If we look at some of the African nations with the largest percent of their diet being indigenous to Africa, look at what we see:

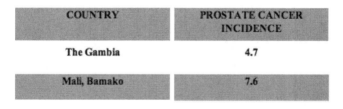

COUNTRY	PROSTATE CANCER INCIDENCE
The Gambia	4.7
Mali, Bamako	7.6

Source: IARC Scientific Publication No. 155. "Cancer Incidence in Five Continents," Vol. 8 Edited by D.M. Parkin. p.633.

Compare these rates with U.S. rates exceeding 200 men per 100,000 population. It would appear that something is differentially causing prostate cancer in African-American men in the United States. I strongly believe that it is dairy consumption that is preferentially affecting African-American men in the United States and other Western countries. It is in these Western countries that dairy products are consumed.

The third jeopardy affecting black men in the U.S. is the biological process, which explains the increasing rates of prostate cancer as one moves from the south to the north. If you guessed that is involves levels of vitamin D, you would be correct.

The brothers Garland point out in their 2006 article that: "Vitamin D status differs by latitude and race, with residents of the northeastern states and individuals with more skin pigmentation (African–Americans) being at increased risk of deficiency."[9] The authors looked at several different types of cancers, including prostate, and concluded that the risk of such cancer could be reduced by adequate supplementation with vitamin D.[10]

The fourth jeopardy affecting black men in the United States and elsewhere is what is known as genetic polymorphisms. This is a technical term for mutations in our DNA. The specific mutations that I am talking about are those in the genes that make the enzymes CYP1A1 and CYP1B1.[11] Specifically there is a form of CYP1B1 that is more active in African-Americans than Caucasians.[12] Remember that CYP1B1 can create the "bad" estrogen? The ratio of this enzyme in African-Americans to Caucasians is approximately 1.7.[13] The ratio of prostate cancer in African-Americans to Caucasians is also approximately 1.6. I do not believe this is a coincidence.

Before I conclude this chapter, I want to put to rest the myth that African-American men can't get prostate cancer from dairy because they may not be consuming it due to their high rate of lactose intolerance. Lactose is one of the sugars contained in milk, and it may not be digested in some individuals because they were born with a deficiency of the enzyme to digest it known as *lactase*. This deficiency can lead to bloating and diarrhea.

It has been estimated that as many as 75 percent-100 percent of African-Americans may have lactose intolerance.[14] Suarez and scientists found that lactose intolerant individuals could tolerate two cups of milk a day without troublesome symptoms.[15] The National Dairy Council reports that "A consumer-based survey found that only 24 percent of African-Americans considered themselves to be lactose intolerant."[16] This means that even if an African-American were to eat some dairy products, it is unlikely that they would have troublesome symptoms. At a prostate disparity conference held in Washington, D.C. and at a famous university I have heard scientists looking at prostate cancer causes say that dairy cannot be the cause because African-Americans can't tolerate dairy and do not eat it. Maybe the first part of their research programs should be to ask African-Americans what I ask them: do you eat dairy products? Their answer is almost always yes. *This excuse must be abandoned immediately!*

So there you have it! The increased risk of prostate cancer in African-American men in the United States and Western countries occurs because of their skin color and the adaptive mechanisms that allow their children to mature more rapidly. Some African-American men and women are genetically predisposed to breast and prostate cancer because they more effectively convert consumed estrogens into the "bad" estrogen C16. This is because of an overactive CYP1B1 enzyme. All these effects occur because Americans and other Western societies consume a dairy-rich diet. Humans are just not adapted to eat dairy from cows! Read on, and let me show you how modern dairy practices have affected the milk you consume.

What You Should Have Learned From This Chapter:

1. African-American men have a much higher risk of prostate cancer than their Caucasian counterparts in Western countries.

2. African-American men have lower levels of IGF-1 binding protein three than their Caucasian counterparts.

3. African-American men have higher levels of PSA than their Caucasian counterparts.

4. Lower levels of IGF-1 binding protein three and higher levels of PSA increase an African-American man's risk of prostate cancer.

5. Lower levels of IGF-1 binding protein three and higher levels of PSA are an adaptive mechanism to make a child mature quickly.

6. African-American men and women have lower levels of serum Vitamin D. This predisposes them to a higher risk of prostate and breast cancer.

7. African-American men have defective mutations in the enzymes CYP1A1and CYP1B1 that cause the ratio of "good" to "bad" estrogens to be unfavorable.

8. Most African-American men and women tolerate dairy-product consumption very well.

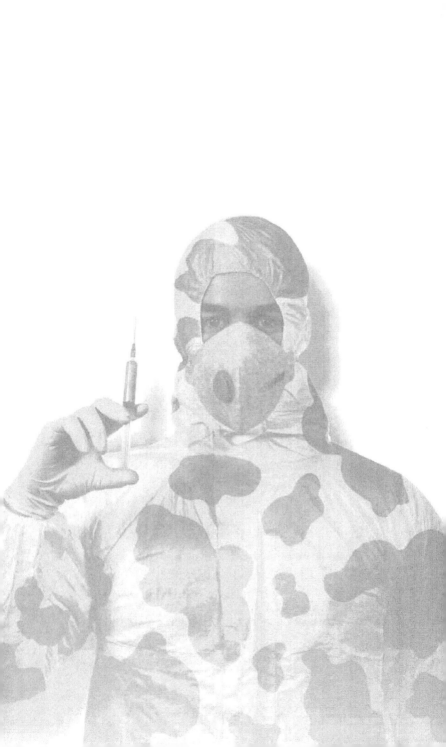

PROSTATE CANCER: THE EPIGENETICS

The incidence rates of prostate cancer in younger men are increasing (see Figure One). This would imply that the average age of men developing prostate cancer is decreasing, and the rate at which younger men are getting prostate cancer is increasing. This same phenomenon has also been observed in women with breast cancer. These mechanisms have been poorly understood and blamed on vague environmental factors influencing the development of these cancers.

An alternate and scientifically sound explanation does exist for this situation. The process is called *epigenetic mutation*. This process involves a reversible change in genes that prevent cancer. This epigenetic process causes normal cells to be transformed into cancer cells.

The epigenetic process acts by turning off or on biochemical switches that allow genes to work. Genes that prevent cancer are called suppressor genes. Genes that cause cancer are called oncogenes. All humans and animals have them. In the cancer-causing process, genes that prevent cancer (suppressor genes) are being turned off, and genes that cause cancer (oncogenes) are being turned on. These on and off switching mechanisms are known as epigenetic mutations. These epigenetic changes can be transmitted through sperm or eggs. This means that anything affecting epigenetic changes can be transmitted to your children and grandchildren. Since most cancers are believed to be caused by these epigenetic changes, this would mean that something in the environment is causing them.

☠

This across generation transmission means that whatever the cause of the epimutational or on and off switching event in your grandparents or parents, it is likely being passed on through the generations. In a more visual explanation, if IGF-1 and estrogens in dairy can cause an epimutational event in a grandparent or parent, it could possibly increase the child's risk of developing prostate or breast cancer. I learned through a physician friend recently that the youngest person with breast cancer is an eleven-year-old!

Figure One: Prostate cancer incidence 1975–2004 for African-American men, Caucasian men, and all men.[2]

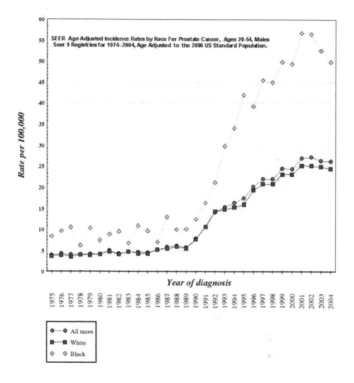

SEER Age Adjusted Incidence Rates by Race For Prostate Cancer, Ages 20-54, Males Seer 9 Registries for 1974–2004, Age Adjusted to the 2000 US Standard Population.

Rate per 100,000

Year of diagnosis

- ● All races
- ■ White
- ◇ Black

Source: SEER Statistical Data Base, U.S. Government. "Prostate cancer incidence 1975–2004 for African-American men, Caucasian men, and all men," (2008) http://www.seer.cancer.gov/

To understand the epimutational (switching) processes, it is necessary to explain and separate this from mutational events. A mutation is a permanent change in your DNA. A mutation is nonreversible. There are certain cancers that are caused by permanent mutations, and most of these mutations are in suppressor genes. It is because of these permanent mutations that a small percentage of prostate, breast, and other cancers would include nonenvironmental (inherited) forms of prostate cancer and other malignancies.

The fact is that most forms of prostate cancer do not fit any one form of inheritable pattern, and the best that can be said is that there is significant heterogeneity (mixed pattern of inheritance).[3] The reason that no one pattern of inheritance fits best is explained by the fact that the cause of prostate cancer is influenced by external environmental causes (diet), which results in reversible epimutational changes in the genes of prostate and likely breast cells.

To understand the difference between mutational and epimutational events, I will briefly outline both processes.

When a cell divides and makes an exact replica of itself, the process is called *mitosis.* During this process, the DNA of the cell, which consists of two parallel strands of chemicals twisted into the so-called double helix, splits apart, and the cell machinery replaces each complimentary chemical with another. If all goes well, the chemicals are replaced in the proper sequence. If the chemicals are identical to their predecessors, then an identical replica of the DNA is produced. If a chemical is not replaced with an identical twin, then a mutation has occurred. This new mutated DNA is permanent. This new but abnormal DNA will be subsequently replicated in all other daughter cells. If this resulting abnormal DNA is now part of a defective suppressor gene, a cancer could develop. This is demonstrated in Figure Five.

Figure Two : Mitosis.[4]

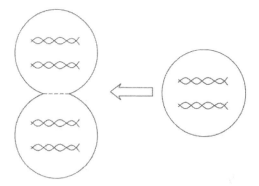

Figure Two: A mother cell divides to reproduce two identical daughter cells.

Figure Three: DNA strand splitting during mitosis.[5]

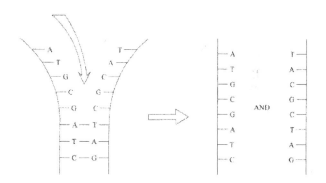

DNA during mitosis: DNA splits into two strands as demonstrated in Figure Three. These strands are comprised of chemicals called nucleic acids and are named adenine (A), cytosine (C), guanine (G), and thymine (T). During normal cell division, the now split individual DNA strands have their individual nucleic acids paired again, resulting in two identical daughter strands of the original DNA as demonstrated in Figure Four.

Figure Four: Two identical strands of DNA.[6]

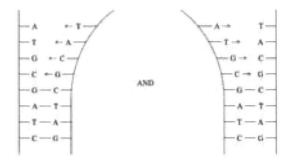

Figure Five: Incorrect DNA match.[7]

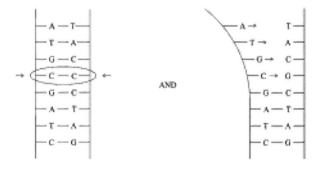

Figure Four: If a nucleic acid match is incorrectly made, such as the cytosine-cytosine example demonstrated above, then a mutation has now occurred. This is a permanent change in the gene, and this will be passed on to subsequent generations. If it occurs in a suppressor gene, a cancer could develop.

The total collections of genes that operate us as human beings are known as the *human genome*. The function of genes is to make proteins. Genes can be turned on and off. This process is the way that a cell can use the DNA to manufacture the proteins that allow it to function normally or to stop the manufacture of particular proteins that could be harmful. Since cells need normal proteins to function, then it is necessary that the DNA and healthy cells be protected. There are particular genes that guard our cells from passing on defective genes to the next generation. One particular gene is known as the p53 gene. I mentioned the operation of this gene in a previous chapter. Some scientists have called this gene the "guardian of the genome." This gene is so called because it is able to recognize defective DNA or defective cells and cause them to die. The malfunction of this gene can lead to dangerous consequences, such as cancer. This p53 gene would be considered a major suppressor gene. Remember suppressor genes are so called because they help prevent cancerous cells from developing.

The process of gene turn-on and turn-off is used by normal cell function. If an abnormal off or on change is not recognized as such by the p53suppressor gene, this failure could result in loss of other protective genes. A broad pattern of suppressor gene turn-off could result in cancer. This is what we see in the so-called heat maps, a process described later in this book.

One of the ways that a gene can be switched on or off is through attachment of a methyl group to the portions of a gene called *CpG islands*. A methyl group is a carbon atom with three hydrogen atoms attached to it (CH3). These CPG islands are basically cytosine(C)-guanine(G) couplets strung together like railroad cars. The P stands for phosphate. These islands are used as one of the switching devices to turn a gene on or off.

These islands occur in what are known as promoter regions of genes because they promote the action of that gene. If all the CpG couplets get a methyl group attached to them, a process called hypermethylation has been said to occur. Hypermethylation generally results in a gene being turned off.

Figure Six: Methyl group.[8]

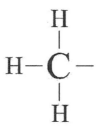

Figure Six: CpG islands unmethylated.[9]

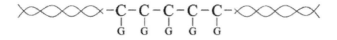

Figure Six: A segment of a gene showing the couplet CpG islands in the unmethylated state. This gene is in the "on" position.

Figure Eight: CpG islands methylated.[10]

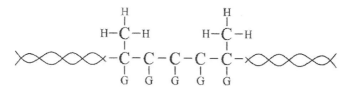

Figure Eight: A gene with a methylated CpG island. It is turned "off."

The process of turning a gene on and off comprises the phenomenon known as *epimutation*. As I mentioned before, one of the genes involved in preventing cancers in humans is the p53 gene.[11] It produces proteins that cause abnormal cells to die. Hypermethylation (gene turned off) of segments of this gene have been identified in the p53 genes of human cells in cancer of the prostate, breast, ovary, and endometrium.[12]

Hypermethylation (epimutation) of the p53 and other genes that prevent cells from dying is likely the cause behind most human cancers. If a cell cannot die, it then becomes immortal and has formed a collection of cells that are now tumorous. The genes that prevent us from getting cancer, such as p53, are called *suppressor genes*. Their hypermethylation (turn off) is responsible for the loss of cancer protection. This could account for the variable inheritance pattern for prostate cancer previously described.[13] Let us take a breather and discuss this important concept.

Let us say that your father had prostate cancer but you did not. This could occur because he ate dairy. You did not eat dairy and turned your protective (suppressor) genes back on and you did not get prostate cancer.

If you ate dairy too and got cancer, it would most likely be because you inherited turned off genes from your father. Your cancer would seem like it was inherited. This is the strange pattern that geneticists struggle with. They cannot pin any pattern of inheritance to prostate cancer. This is why: if you eat dairy you may get prostate cancer, and if you do not eat dairy, you may not get prostate cancer! Remember this important fact: almost all cancers are epigenetic (environmental) and not genetic. This means that your environment is causing your cancer. The environment does so by turning off genes that are designed to protect you against cancer. This process is called an epigenetic process because it does not permanently affect your genes. It simply turns them "off." This means that things you ingest in your environment, including dairy products, may be causing your cancers.

Another way to look at this phenomenon is that a gene's activity is like a furnace, its heat intensity being controlled by a thermostat. A gene's activity is controlled by how many of its CpG islands contain methyl groups. This is the same thing as stating how much it is methylated. Methylation is the thermostat. It controls how many and to what extent a gene is turned "off." Methylation (turn-off) of the suppressor genes that prevent cancer can be looked at using biochemical techniques. These techniques use chemicals to detect how many methyl groups have been attached to the CpG islands. Remember the more methyl groups attached, the more a gene is turned "off." A gene can be completely turned off like a light switch or partially turned off. The partial turn-off would be like using a dimmer on the light switch. The pictures developed by the technique of looking at methyl groups attached to protective genes are known as a heat maps.

Heat maps have been developed to look at various suppressor genes that control prevention of cancer. Chung has published such a heat map for some of these genes and the respective cancers that they were found in.[14] I must point out that all human cells contain the same suppressor genes. It becomes an interesting exercise to see what suppressor genes are turned off in certain cancers. Chart One is the *heat map*, which they published for prostate cancer. They are called heat maps because they are color coded by the degree of methylation where white means fully turned on (protective) and red would be fully turned off. Since red means a protective gene is fully "turned off," a high risk of cancer developing is present. The resulting shades of pink and red look like the various colors of red in a furnace or fire. Remember, since this book is printed in gray scale, what would normally be red is dark gray. Dark gray would mean a gene is turned off. Remember white is good. Dark gray is bad, and light gray is somewhere in between. Light gray would imply that you are on the way to turning that protective gene "off."

Chart One: Prostate cancer heat map.[15]

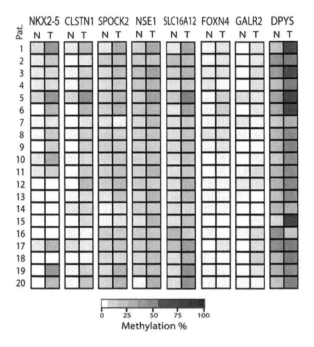

Chart One: Chung W. et al., "Identification of Novel Tumor Markers in Prostate, Colon, and Breast Cancer by Unbiased Methylation,"Profiling. PLoS ONE. 3 (2008) http://www.PloS one. org. (The genes that were studied are listed at the top, and the degree of heat (in shades of gray) represents the degree of methylation.)

Other authors have looked at the turn-off process (epigenetic mutation) in prostate cancer. Kang looked at higher Gleason score prostate cancer (advanced) versus low Gleason score (early) and found a higher degree of turned-off suppressor genes in the more advanced cancers. It was the conclusion of their investigation that CpG-island methylation (turn-off) was a frequent

ROBERT BIBB, MD

event in prostate cancer development and that perhaps the process of measuring the degree of methylation could serve as a marker for advanced prostate cancer.[16]

Ellinger and his research team looked at gene hypermethylation (increased methyl group attachment to CpG islands) in prostate cancer cell lines and concluded that methylation of CpG islands could be helpful in diagnosing prostate cancer and may be used to predict early biochemical reoccurrence after radical prostatectomy.[17] Remember that attachment of methyl groups to CpG islands is known as methylation, and it is the same thing as turning a gene off.

One of the most important points that I want to make about an epigenetic mutation (turn-off of genes) is that it is inheritable and potentially reversible. This means you may be able to turn your protective genes back on and perhaps make a cancer die. This also means that you can pass the changes on to the next generation. Nephew et al. makes this statement clear in a 2003 paper by stating: "Because of their (in)heritable nature, hypermethylated CpG islands leave 'molecular footprints' in evolving cancer cells and can be used as molecular markers to reconstruct epigenetic progression during tumorigenesis."[18] In other words, by looking at heat maps we should be able to track how a noncancerous cell becomes a cancerous one.

Now, imagine the impact if a commonly ingested material were to hypermethylate (turn-off) certain genes in pregnant women and then predispose the unborn human to cancer later in life!

Imprinting is a term used as a synonym for gene turn-on or gene turn-off. Perinatal means around the time of birth.

In an article entitled "*Perinatal Imprinting by Estrogen and Adult Prostate Disease,*" Olie Söder writes,

> One of the major conceptual novelties in human medicine emerging during the last two decades is the fetal-origin hypothesis, challenging our traditional view on the pathogenesis of common chronic disorders. This hypothesis originally put forward by Barker and other scientists (1), states that prenatal events, mainly of nutritional and metabolic nature are memorized ("imprinted") by the developing organism and, if inappropriate for the postnatal situation, may result in the development of diseases during adult age.[19]

Think about this for a moment. What Barker is saying is that what a woman eats before birth may affect her child. What he is talking about here is not killing the child by consumption of a poison but turning on or off certain genes. He is talking about epigenetic events occurring in the unborn child that will affect it later in life. What he is describing here is that which I am greatly concerned about. He is describing the key event about which this book centers. He is describing the events that I believe are causing the epidemic of breast and prostate cancer. He is describing how I believe that ingestion of dairy products through estrogens and IGF-1 are causing important protective genes to be turned off, resulting in cancer in the U.S. population!

Söder's article continues to comment about a study by Omoto and fellow scientists in which pregnant rats exposed to an estrogenic compound gave birth to male rats predisposed to prostate cancer later in life and that this imprinting (epigenetic events) was caused through the effects of estrogen receptor alpha.[20] Remember that imprinting of genes, epigenetic changes in genes, and gene "turn-off" are the same event. They mean that genes that protect against cancer and are called suppressor genes are being "turned off."

Let me restate what you just read: *pregnant rats ingesting estrogenic compounds during pregnancy resulted in their male offspring developing prostate cancer later in life!*

The estrogenic compounds used in the cited experiments were not milk, but dairy does contain powerful estrogens. Now you can see why I am worried. One of the estrogenic compounds used in Omoto's study was bisphenol A, a material used to make plastic.[21] It is a so-called *xeno-estrogen. Xeno* is Greek for "like." These xeno-estrogenic compounds are typically less strong than natural estrogens. If we are going to have "conversations" about plastics causing prostate cancer, then let us add milk and milk products to the discussion.

I have further anxiety when I look at the rate of change in incidence of prostate cancer over time. The statistical data that the U.S. government collects and then provides for all to review is "age-adjusted." *Age adjustment* means that the increase in incidence rate that we are looking at is not caused by an aging population. Now let us return to the graphs of incidence of prostate cancer in men who are less than age fifty versus time.

Figure Nine: Prostate cancer incidence 1975–2004 for African-American men, Caucasian men, and all men.[2]

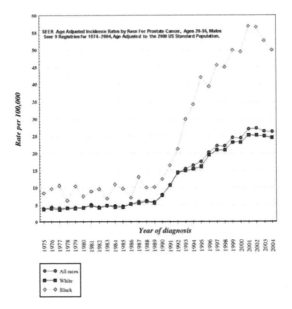

Source: Figure Nine: SEER Statistical Data Base, U.S. government. "Prostate cancer incidence 1975–2004 for African-American men, Caucasian men, and all men," (2008) http://www.seer.cancer.gov/

Look at the overall rates and then concentrate on the incidence rate over time for African-American men. This curve approaches infinity. *These curves would imply that something is causing an accumulative effect over time and that this process is much worse for African-American men.* Could this effect be an imprinting change in genes for prostate cancer being passed from generation to generation? It is very possible that this is the process that we are looking at. What if this was caused by a common food(s) substance we are all ingesting? A thought like this could keep you awake at night.

This accumulative process is similar to the curve you see for compound interest. The accumulation there is money. The accumulative material in the incidence curves for prostate cancer over time is, I suspect, turned off suppressor genes. I have outlined this principle in Appendix G.

Another mechanism that could assist in the development of cancer of the breast and prostate is the process by which the DNA of the cells is changed through interaction other estrogen metabolites called quinones.[23] This process would also likely result in mutations that could also be transmitted to the next generation.

What You Should Have Learned From This Chapter:

1. A mutation is a permanent change in your genes(s).

2. An epimutation is a reversible change in your gene(s).

3. Hypermethylation (epimutation) of a gene will usually turn it off.

4. Most prostate cancer is due to epimutational (turn-off) events.

5. Estrogen exposure in pregnancy may imprint (turn off certain genes) male offspring for a higher risk of prostate cancer later in life.

6. A serious concern is developing regarding potential (in)heritable changes in genes accumulating intergenerationally (between generations), resulting in an ever-increasing rate of prostate cancer.

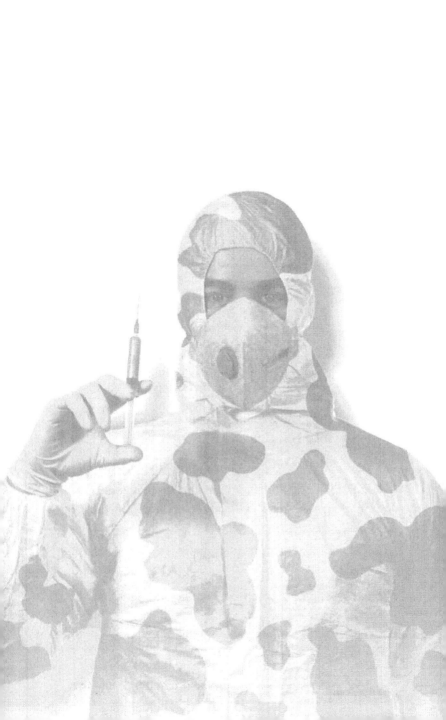

MODERN DAIRY PRACTICES

I am going to discuss in this chapter the modern dairy practices designed to increase milk yield from dairy cows and what effect that this has had on the milk composition. I will also discuss some of the processing techniques that have led to increased concentrations of the hormones and proteins of concern. I will also elaborate on some of the marketing techniques that, I believe, have placed the consumer at risk of cancer development. These marketing techniques are promoting products that contain the hormones and proteins mentioned above. *Let me be very clear about the fact that cows naturally secrete all the hormones and proteins that may be increased in their milk by the modern dairy practices discussed.*

The main purpose of using hormones in dairy herds is simple: to increase the yield of milk in relationship to what cows are fed. This keeps the cost of maintaining dairy herds at the most efficient level for milk production.

There are a number of hormones that cows are given, such as estrogens, progesterone, and, of course, growth hormones. The main use of most hormones is in cattle for beef consumption. These hormones definitely increase the natural estrogens and growth hormones left in the tissue of beef after slaughter. These residual levels are higher when compared to cattle in which they are not used. The residual hormones left in beef tissue are low when we compare these levels to hormones secreted in milk in both untreated and treated cows. There are two modern-day farming methods that have increased the levels of hormones naturally contained in cow's milk. They are the technique of keeping cows pregnant almost continuously and the use of externally administered hormones.

The main hormone administered to cows to increase milk production is what is known as *recombinant bovine growth hormone* (rBGH). It is synthetically manufactured using bacteria. The structure of the rBGH is meant to mimic the natural bovine growth hormone known as *bovine somatotropin* (rBGH); however, it is not identical to bovine somatotropin but differs by one amino acid at the end of the molecule. Both natural and synthetic rBGH attach to receptors on the surface of target cells and mainly exert their influence by stimulation of the production of insulin-like growth factor one (IGF-1).

The main synthetic rBGH used in U.S. dairy herds is manufactured by Monsanto Corporation under the trademark name Posilac®. The use of Posilac® in U.S. dairy cattle was approved in 1994 by the Federal Drug Administration (FDA). The claim by Monsanto is that the use of Posilac® can increase milk production by an average of 10 percent over 300 days.[2]

The approval of Posilac® was not without controversy. In an article published online and entitled *"Whistleblowers, Threats and Bribes: a Short History of Genetically Engineered Bovine Growth Hormones,"* Jeffrey Smith describes the controversial introduction of rBGH into U.S. dairy herds.[3, 4]

Several scientific investigators who were involved in the original evaluation of rBGH were concerned about the science or procedures involved in the evaluation of rBGH.[5] Smith contends in his article that these individuals were either pressured to leave or were demoted. Other concerned scientists at the FDA, Smith notes, were concerned enough to write an anonymous letter to members in the Congress stating that they had fear about giving an honest opinion about the use of rBGH because of fear of retaliation. Even more interesting is the fact that the FDA employee who wrote the opinion about not labeling milk from rBGH dairy herds had previously been employed by Monsanto as a researcher on Posilac®.[6]

With enough intrigue and controversy to make a great novel, Posilac® was approved by the FDA for use in dairy cows in 1994. Despite its use in the U.S., rBGH has not been approved in Japan, Australia, New Zealand, Canada, or the twenty-seven nation members of the European Union.[7]

Beyond the concerns of alteration of the content of milk produced from cows given rBGH, there has been enough evidence over time to be worried about the health of the dairy cows. There has been reported an increase risk of mastitis (udder irritation or infection), substantial reductions in fertility, and lameness.[8]

Science supports the fact that rBGH, itself, is not likely harmful to humans, but what it does to milk and the tissue of beef has raised great concern.[9] As I pointed previously, beef tissue does contain residues of estrogens and insulin-like growth factors, but the majority of these harmful hormones and proteins in a Western diet are obtained from dairy consumption.

Dr. Margaret Miller was originally involved in Posilac® research at Monsanto Corporation and then was later employed at the FDA. While in the employment of the FDA, she wrote a first draft paper about the evaluation of Posilac®. In this article she cited a scientific paper that stated that IGF-1 in the milk of cows treated with rBGH was not outside the values of normal from untreated cows.[10] Although her assertion seems true at first glance, you must look at how this interpretation could be viewed as a favorable presentation of the actual facts.

Anytime statistical data is collected from a population, whether this is humans or cows, a variation in the data collected will range from a low value to a high value. Typically, the data will fit a bell-shaped curve. This bell-shaped curve is called a *normal distribution*. Let us look at such set of curves generated from a dairy herd given Posilac® and a herd that was free of Posilac®. Daxenberger and colleagues performed such an experiment in 1998, and here is a representation of what they found[11]:

Figure One: Normal distribution curve for IGF-1 in milk from cows given rBGH versus cows not given rBGH.[12]

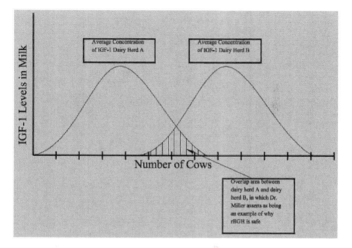

Source: Figure One: Adapted from "Daxenberger and fellow scientists. Increased milk levels of insulin-like growth factor 1 (IGF-1) for the identification of bovine somatotropin (bST) treated cows," Analyst. (1998):2429–35.

From the representation in Figure One, it is obvious that some cows not given rBGH secrete high levels of IGF-1 in their milk, and some cows that were given rBGH secrete low levels of IGF-1; but the mean levels of IGF-1 from herds given rBGH are much higher.[13] The mean is the value obtained from looking at the peak in the curve. This means that if you are drinking milk from cows given rBGH, you are consuming higher levels of IGF-1 than milk from cows not given the growth hormone.[14] You ask: how much higher? From Jeffrey Smith's article, it has been reported that a doubling of

IGF-1, and perhaps as much as 3.6 times as much IGF-1, can occur in cows treated with Posilac®.[15] Remember, the effect of a hormone is magnified many-fold by the secondary messenger system described earlier. This is the bowling ball effect. So a 3.6 times greater level of IGF-1 in milk could mean a many times greater end effect in the body. Untreated cows still secrete the dangerous hormones and proteins. In my opinion, no dairy at the present time is safe. Are the lower levels of hormones and proteins in untreated cows safer? I do not believe this to be true. It just may take you longer to get prostate or breast cancer.

☠

The more complex question of why should you care about higher IGF-1 in your milk is answered by the fact that IGF-1 levels in the bloodstream have been associated with both a higher incidence of prostate cancer and premenopausal breast cancer. I have discussed this phenomenon earlier in this book.

I pointed out early on in this book that prostate cancer incidence started its meteoric rise around 1950, shortly after the discontinuation of exposure of milk to ultraviolet light. I also suggested that this rise in incidence may have occurred because ultraviolet light inactivated IGF-1 by a process called *denaturization*. Denaturization occurs because of interruption of disulfide bonds holding IGF-1 together. The early experiments performed at Clemson University by Dr. Lyndom Larcom suggested that this might be the case.[16]

With the knowledge that rBGH was introduced into dairy herds in the U.S. in 1994, might we expect to see another spike in incidence of prostate cancer and premenopausal breast cancer in children raised on increased levels of IGF-1 in their dairy products?[17] If the history of the appearance of IGF-1 in milk since 1950 is accurate, then this should be the case.

☠

I want to go on record now and state as clearly and loudly as possible that my prediction is that we will see an increase in the incidence of teenage breast cancer and men in their twenties and early thirties developing prostate cancer if elevated levels of IGF-1 are allowed to continue in dairy products by the continued use of rBGH and continued use of "good animal" husbandry techniques that allow significantly elevated levels of estrogens and IGF-1 to be secreted in cows' milk.

Another dairy practice that has increased hormones and proteins in milk has been the use of modern-day feed practices and milking cows while pregnant. Ganmaa points out in an article in 2005 that modern dairy practices are much different than one hundred years ago, when cows were pasture fed. Modern dairy practices include milking cows while pregnant. This practice can increase the levels of estrogens in milk.[8] In fact, Ganmaa asserts in the *Harvard University Gazette* that in the later stages of pregnancy cows can secrete up to 33 times as much estrogen as nonpregnant cows.[9]

Let me now turn to some of the modern-day processing of milk-derived products that the consumer may or may not be aware come from milk. There are the obvious products, such as milk, ice cream, cream, yogurt, and butter. Consumers may not think about whole milk powders; nonfat dry-milk powders, butter oils; and the milk protein concentrates that include whey, casein, and other protein concentrates. Did you know, for example, that lactoferrin is a milk-derived protein? It has antimicrobial properties and is approved by the FDA to spray on beef carcasses as a preservative.[20]

Other dairy-derived products that reach our palates include cream in light and heavy whipping creams, half and half, sour cream, and previously mentioned caseins. Caseins are the fat-soluble proteins derived from milk and will be processed and marketed as ammonium caseinates, calcium caseinates, casein hydrolysates, magnesium caseinates, paracaseinates, potassium caseinate, rennet casein, sodium caseinate, and zinc caseinate. These can be included in cheeses marketed as vegetarian.[21]

Additional dairy-derived products include the curd from milk. It is the precipitated material from milk used to make cheese. It is used also in cottage cheese. Lactoalbumin is a dairy-derived protein from whey and is used as an emulsifying agent. Lactoglobulin is a whey protein that may be seen in sports beverages.[22]

Colustrum is the material produced by the cow mammary gland for the first few days after birth of their calves. It is used in numerous products, including nutraceuticals.[23]

One product in particular has me greatly concerned, and that is whey protein powders. They are marketed as products that are useful in losing weight and building muscle. This is certainly likely to be an accurate claim. Whey is the liquid portion of the milk left when casein is precipitated out to make cheese. What remains as whey are the water-soluble materials. These include

IGF-1 conjugated estrogens (water-soluble estrogens) and other water-soluble proteins. This material can be concentrated further by filtration processes. The processed dry whey can have very high levels of IGF-1 and estrogens. When individuals use concentrated whey products for weight loss and muscle build-up, they are being exposed to high levels of IGF-1 and estrogens. Remember IGF-1 and estrogens are the main biochemicals thought to be linked to the development of prostate cancer! Do not consume whey!

Marketing dairy products through the use of famous personalities with milk rings around their mouth has become an iconic association with the benefits of milk. I am reminded of the front page cover of a magazine that deals with women's issues with cancer. On the cover was a picture of a prominent folk singer, and inside was a great article in which she discussed her bout with cancer. There was also an ad of this performer with the milk ring around her mouth. It made me feel sick inside to wonder if she knew about what was in her dairy. I did write a letter to her through the editors, but I never heard back from her.

I have also seen ads stating that you need calcium from milk to make your bones strong. There is no doubt that you need calcium to accomplish this task, but you do not need it from milk. Let me address this controversy in the next chapter.

What You Should Have Learned From This Chapter:

1. Cows naturally secrete all the hormones implicated in causing breast and prostate cancer.

2. Recombinant bovine growth hormone (rBGH) is known as Posilac®.

3. Posilac® is given to dairy cows to increase milk production.

4. Controversy surrounds the introduction of Posilac® into U.S. dairy herds.

4. Posilac® dramatically increases the amount of IGF-1 secreted into milk.

5. Cows are kept pregnant to increase milk production.

6. Cows secrete high levels of estrogens into their milk when they are pregnant.

7. You are reminded that IGF-1 and estrogens in milk have been implicated in the development of prostate and premenopausal breast cancers.

8. There are sources of dairy that you might not be aware exist in your food.

9. Whey protein contains high levels of IGF-1.

CALCIUM FROM DAIRY: THE MYTH

When I talk with my patients about avoiding dairy products, the most common question I hear is "How do I get my calcium?" or "What do I give my child so they can get their calcium?" These patients are really meaning to ask "How do I get calcium other than from milk?" The dairy advertisements have done a good job convincing us that milk is a necessity for such an important nutrient. Let me convince you that dairy is also not necessary for this purpose either.

One of the developing controversies regarding the use of dairy in the neonatal period is the possibility of imprinting the child for a higher risk of prostate or breast cancer later in life. I discussed this concern in an earlier chapter. It would then be a logical question to ask

"How do I get the calcium needed to make my child's bones strong and reduce my chance of osteoporosis and cancer later in life?"

Now let me answer that question by taking you logically through the evidence to show you that dairy is not necessary for the calcium our bodies need. The first place to start is to look at what amount of calcium we actually need. From the *Journal of Pediatrics* in 1978, the following recommendations are listed:

Table One: Calcium intake recommendation versus age.[2]

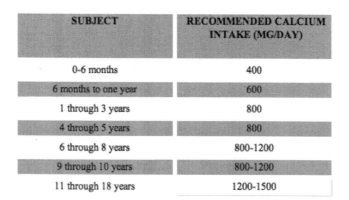

SUBJECT	RECOMMENDED CALCIUM INTAKE (MG/DAY)
0-6 months	400
6 months to one year	600
1 through 3 years	800
4 through 5 years	800
6 through 8 years	800-1200
9 through 10 years	800-1200
11 through 18 years	1200-1500

Table One: "Calcium Requirement of Infants, Children and Adolescents. (Committee on Nutrition)"Pediatrics. 104 (1999):1152–57.

The National Academy of Sciences has established the following calcium levels for adults:

Table Two: Recommended calcium intake for adults

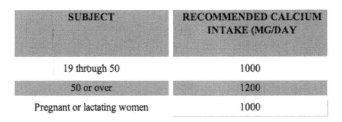

SUBJECT	RECOMMENDED CALCIUM INTAKE (MG/DAY
19 through 50	1000
50 or over	1200
Pregnant or lactating women	1000

Source: Table Two: Harvard School of Public Health (2008) http://www.hsph.harvard.edu/nutritionsource/calcium.htmililiters

Calcium is certainly necessary to allow normal bone development and is also required for other physiologic processes to proceed normally within our cells. I take a strong stance that it is not only dangerous to use milk to obtain your calcium, but it is also unnecessary to obtain it from this source.

Let me start with some of the scientific evidence to support my claim. A report in 1997 revealed the results of 77,761 women ages thirty-four to fifty-nine, who were followed over a twelve-year period starting in 1980. This large group of women had never used calcium supplements and was interviewed regarding their dietary intake. The researchers were investigating whether higher intakes of calcium from foods or milk reduced the chance of hip or forearm fracture. The conclusion of the study was that: "These data do not support the hypothesis that higher intake of milk or other food sources of calcium by adult women protects against hip fracture or forearm fracture."[3] This study would appear to debunk the myth that dairy consumption reduces osteoporosis in women. You might be thinking, *Sure, for adults dairy might not be necessary, but my child's bones aren't formed yet.* Have I got some surprising information for you!

In a seminal paper published in 2005, Lanou and other scientists looked at all the available published papers that studied the effects of dairy products and total dietary calcium intake on bone strength in children and young adults. In all, fifty-eight papers were reviewed, and the conclusion of the authors was that there is little evidence to support that recommending an increased dairy diet promotes bone strength in children or adolescents.[4]

Dr. Lanou does point out that sunlight and physical activity have the strongest influence on bone health in children. She does recommend getting adequate amounts of calcium from fruits and vegetables.[5] As a dermatologist, I would replace sunlight with adequate oral levels of vitamin D3, which is otherwise known as cholecalciferol.

In a young child or a newborn baby that is not being nursed, adequate levels of calcium can be obtained from soy-based infant formulas. Soy-based formulas are usually supplemented with a form of calcium called *calcium carbonate.* This is the type of calcium used in antacids and most calcium supplements. Sheikh determined that this form of calcium was as well absorbed as the calcium in cow's milk.[6] In a study published in 2005, Zhao and his collaborators confirmed the previous study by noting that the bioavailability of calcium from supplemented soy milk was the same as that from cow's milk.[7]

A great reference source for foods containing calcium is the *USDA National Nutrient Database for Standard Reference, Release* 17. This reference lists the calcium content of various food items. Examples of such foods are listed in Table Three.

Table Three: Various foods and calcium content

FOOD DESCRIPTION	CALCIUM CONTENT IN MG.
Cooked collards-one cup	357
Canned spinach-one cup	272
Cooked soybeans-one cup	261
Cooked turnip greens	249
Bread crumbs-one cup	218
Cooked white beans-one cup	191
Sub sandwich 6" cold cuts	189
Canned salmon-3 oz	181
Cooked beet greens	164
Slice of cornbread	162
Tomato soup-one cup	159
Cooked cabbage	158
Egg and sausage biscuit	155
Tofu one serving	133
Cooked Okra	123
Peanut butter-one tbsp	7

Source: Table Three: From *USDA National Nutrient Database for Standard Reference, Release* 17.

I intentionally added peanut butter to show that it is not a good source of calcium. If there is a concern about how much calcium can be obtained from foods, the FDA required food label can be a great resource. I have added an example from the FDA's Web site.[8]

Nutrition Facts

Serving Size ½ cup (114g)
Servings Per Container 4

Amount Per Serving

Calories 90   Calories from Fat 30

% Daily Value*

Total Fat 3g	**5%**
Saturated Fat 0g	**0%**
Cholesterol 0mg	**0%**
Sodium 300mg	**13%**
Total Carbohydrate 13g	**4%**
Dietary Fiber 3g	**12%**
Sugars 3g	
Protein 3g	

Vitamin A 80%	•	Vitamin C 60%
Calcium 4%	•	Iron 4%

* Percent Daily Values are based on a 2,000
calorie diet. Your daily values may be higher
or lower depending on your calorie needs:

	Calories:	2,000	2,500
Total Fat	Less than	65g	80g
Sat Fat	Less than	20g	25g
Cholesterol	Less than	300mg	300mg
Sodium	Less than	2,400mg	2,400mg
Total Carbohydrate		300g	375g
Dietary Fiber		25g	30g

Calories per gram:
Fat 9 • Carbohydrate 4 • Protein 4

Source: Figure One: "FDA nutrition label," (2008) http://www.fda.gov/Food/LabelingNutrition/default.htm.[9]

The required FDA food label, as demonstrated in Figure One, will give the reader the percentage of the recommended daily allowance of calcium for an adult.[10]

I hope that I have convinced you that you do not need to get your calcium from dairy. While we are on the subject of diet, let me show you in the next chapter what levels of hormones and protein hormones you are ingesting in a typical dairy diet.

What You Should Have Learned From This Chapter:

1. A certain amount of calcium is necessary and is a function of age.

2. You do not need dairy to get your calcium.

3. There are alternative sources of calcium, no matter what age.

THE AMERICAN GROCERY CART:

Your Toasted Cheese Sandwich

Remember the nursery rhyme?

Little Miss Muffet

Sat on her Tuffet (a small stool)

Eating her curds and whey

Along came a spider

Who sat down beside her

And frightened Miss Muffet away

When I was a child, I remember reciting the first version of the rhyme. I had no idea what a tuffet, whey, or curds (casein) were at that time, and I suspect that this was also true of my young classmates. I am naturally assuming that people would be aware of the obvious dairy products to avoid, such as milk, cheese, and butter, etc, but the "hidden" dairy materials are less obvious. I want to talk about the curds (casein) and whey used in many food products that may not be not considered as "dairy" by the consuming public.

I had an interesting encounter in my office recently that led me to believe that most of my adult patients may not know what whey or casein is. One of my patients had recently been treated for a brain tumor at the renowned medical institution at M. D. Anderson hospital in Houston, Texas. During his inpatient stay, he was asked to sit in on a nutrition class for cancer victims. He was told during this lecture to avoid whey. When he returned home, he did as he was told and became a label reader to avoid this whey material. He also did some research and found out that whey is derived from milk. He then thought it odd that he was not told to avoid dairy products. Remember, he was given the whey avoidance message by a trained health professional. It became obvious to me that most people would not be aware of what curds and whey are and, therefore, would not understand their dangerous composition and consumptive consequences.

Join me now as I take you through the information on these interesting derivatives of milk.

Whey is the name given to the water-soluble portion of milk that is left behind when casein (curds) are precipitated out to make cheese. Whey used to be discarded as a waste material, until the dairy industry learned that they could take out most or all of the water and develop a market for this material. Whey is not one compound but consists of a number of different protein molecules. In a condensed form it is very sticky and can be used as a binding and thickening agent in many food products. It can also impart a creamy consistency to certain non-dairy items, including buttery margarines.

One the many water-soluble molecules in milk and whey is our old nemesis: IGF-1.

Since whey is typically condensed by taking the water out, the IGF-1 concentration in whey-based material can increase. Remember, the previous chapter on IGF-1 explains how this molecule stimulates estrogen receptors alpha to develop on prostate tissue. Remember also, increasing levels of IGF-1 in the bloodstream of men and premenopausal women are associated with increasing incidence of prostate cancer and premenopausal breast cancer respectively. How much can it be concentrated? This depends on how it is purified and processed.

> Whey protein typically comes in three major forms: concentrate, isolate, and hydrosylate. Whey proteins contain a low level of fat and cholesterol but generally have higher levels of bioactive compounds and carbohydrates in the form of lactose—they are 29–89 percent protein by weight. Isolates are processed to remove the fat and lactose but are usually lower in bioactive compounds. Isolates may be as much as 90 percent plus protein by weight. Both isolates and concentrates are mild

to slightly milky in taste. Hydrosylates are predigested, partially hydrolyzed whey proteins, which consequently are more easily absorbed, but their cost is generally higher. Whey protein hydrosylate also tends to taste quite different than other forms of whey protein. Many find this taste undesirable, but it can be masked when used in beverages.[2]

Hydosylates essentially involve digestion of the protein fractions of whey, including IGF-1. They would not be a significant source of retained and free IGF-1. Isolates are primarily produced by using a process known as *reverse osmosis*. This process uses high pressure to force whey liquid through a membrane to separate the proteins. This process does not involve heat, which would otherwise render the IGF-1 inactive. The isolates are usually treated chemically to remove the fat and would not be exposed to significant thermal trauma.[3] What does all this mean to the consumer? It means that whey materials entering the food chain contain significant amounts of undamaged proteins, such as our killer IGF-1.

As I wandered through the aisles of a local grocery store recently, I was amazed at how many seemingly nondairy products contained whey. They included energy bars, energy drinks, and breads, such as loaf, hamburger, and hot-dog rolls. It was in processed cheese products and potato chip products. In our local mall, the body-building products were loaded with it. It was everywhere!

The biggest question I had as I reviewed these products was: does IGF-1 in whey survive elevated temperatures in the pasteurization process necessary to reduce bacteria and extend shelf like? Does it survive baking intact?

Kaddouri and fellow scientists looked at the survivability of the proteins in whey and whole milk after microwave treatments at various energy levels over varying lengths of time. The times varied up to twenty minutes. They found no more than a 50 percent reduction in the protein fractions.[4] Microwave energy works by exciting water molecules in a substance, and at ground level, the heated products usually reach the boiling point of water at 212°F. Hidalgo and fellow researchers showed that the stability of whey proteins is also dependent on pH and can be modified by the calcium salts used to protect typical commercial whey preparations. They found that 40–90 percent of the whey proteins remained intact with temperatures up to 134°C or 273°F and a pH above zero.[5]

Pasteurizationprocesses use the following FDA guidelines[6]:

Table One: Pasteurization and FDA guidelines.[7]

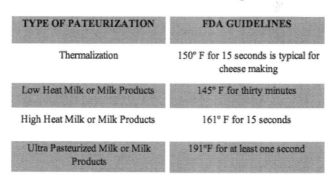

TYPE OF PATEURIZATION	FDA GUIDELINES
Thermalization	150° F for 15 seconds is typical for cheese making
Low Heat Milk or Milk Products	145° F for thirty minutes
High Heat Milk or Milk Products	161° F for 15 seconds
Ultra Pasteurized Milk or Milk Products	191°F for at least one second

Source: Table One: Gourmet Retailer, "Specialty Cheese Series 1-White Heat: Pasteurizationvs. Raw Milk,"(2009) http://www.gourmetretailer.com/gourmetretailer/research/article_display.jsp?vnu_content_id=1000827757

It becomes obvious that the temperatures used to process a significant number of foods containing whey will never become high enough to reach the 273°F to destroy the IGF-1. Most bread products are baked at temperatures in the range of 375°F to 425°F, and at these temperatures most of the whey proteins are likely to become biologically inactive.

What are the actual levels of IGF-1 in whey protein concentrates? This would depend on how pure they are. From Daxenberger and fellow lab researchers in 1998, we learn that the average values for IGF-1 range from 4–35 ng per milliliter in milk from non-rBGH treated dairy herds; however, the high end of the normal range in these herds is the average value for cows treated with recombinant bovine growth hormone (i.e., 35 ng/milliliter).[8] If we look at the weight of milk as roughly as 30 grams per milliliter, then this would turn out to be a value of 35 ng per 30 grams of milk (wet weight). Milk is on the average 87 percent comprised of water.[9] With this fact in mind, the final number we are looking for would be approximately 9 ng of IGF-1 per gram of dried milk. Remember, this is dried milk and not whey. This does not include separation of the whey from the milk and subsequent concentration measures. These measures would only increase the concentration of the IGF-1 in the whey isolates produced for the food industry.

The story on the safety of proteins and hormones in milk products is not over. Grosvenor and fellow researchers noted in their findings that 90 percent of the estrogens in milk are conjugated.[10] *Conjugation* means that these estrogens are water soluble, and if something is water soluble, then it will be in the whey portion of milk.

The water-soluble estrogen in milk is known as estrone sulfate. Wolford's study of estrogen in whey found that the average level of estrone was 3.6 picograms per gram (wet weight).[11] This study was performed in 1979. This was before cows were allowed to be treated with recombinant bovine growth (Posilac®) hormone in 1994. The administration of Posilac® to cows would be expected to increase the estrogen in the whey. We also noted in the chapter on estrogens that Wolford's measurement of these hormones was low compared to other authors. This could be accounted for on the basis of different techniques used. *The most important fact established in the chapter on estrogens was that they likely survive cooking; therefore, estrogens are in your baked goods that also contain whey.*

The curds that little Miss Muffet ate were basically the condensed fat-soluble portion of milk known as *casein.* Casein accounts for more than 80 percent of the proteins contained in milk and cheese.[12] Casein is also found in butter. Caseins are frequently combined with calcium or sodium to promote heat stability and to improve the binding capacity of the proteins. They can then be used as fillers or binding agents in food materials. They would be labeled as *caseinates* such as sodium caseinate, calcium caseinate, or just plain milk protein.[13]

Since casein is the fat-soluble portion of the milk, we would expect to find fat-soluble compounds in this partition of milk. This is in fact true. We find the most potent type of estrogen located in this fraction of milk, and it is 17 beta estradiol. Wolford's study in 1979 confirmed the presence of 17 beta estradiol in milk curd (casein) with the highest level being found in butter.[14]

We have already established that estrogens survive cooking, and therefore, it is obvious that your macaroni and cheese may likely contain estrogens.

The largest use for caseins is in the cheese-making process. In fact, while the consumption of whole milk has declined over the last few decades, the demand for cheese has sky-rocketed. This phenomenon is demonstrated in the following charts.

Figure One: Pounds per capita whole milk over time.[15]

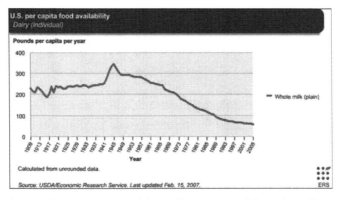

Source: Figure One: United States Department of Agriculture, Economic Research Service, "U.S. Per Capita Food Availability Dairy," (2007) http://www.ers.usda.gov/Search/?qt=Per%20Capita%20Milk%20over%20time.

Figure Two: Poundsper capita cheese over time.[16]

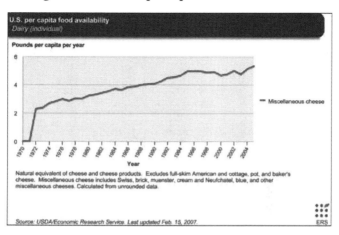

Source: Figure Two: United States Department of Agriculture, Economic Research Service, "U.S. Per Capita Food Availability Dairy," (2007) http://www.ers.usda.gov/Search/?qt=per+capita+cheese+over+time

We can see that the demand for cheese in the United States has increased dramatically. Some individuals have postulated that such a demand may be the increasing desire for Mexican foods that parallels the migration of Spanish speaking cultures to the U.S. and the increasing number of fast food restaurants serving Mexican style foods. Pizza has also become much more popular with the advent of many chain and non-chain stores willing to deliver these cheese-laden carbohydrates.

Whatever the reason for such an increase, you must be aware that you are consuming both IGF-1 and estrogens in the whey- and casein-containing food products that you purchase. If we try to do the math on IGF-1 intake and use the high end of normal in a Posilac® herd, which is 35 nanograms per milliliter and three glasses of milk at 840 milliliters, we get 28 milligrams a day just from the average dairy intake as milk. This compares to the amounts given per day to counteract small stature, which could be levels such as 5 mg per day.[17] I think we should all have concern about this. That includes your toasted cheese sandwich.

☠

Start reading all the labels on the food you purchase!

What You Should Have Learned From This Chapter:

1. Whey is the water-soluble portion of milk.

2. Whey contains IGF-1.

3. Whey contains the water-soluble estrogen: estrone sulfate.

4. Casein is the fat-soluble portion of milk.

5. Casein contains the fat-soluble and most potent estrogen: 17 beta estradiol.

6. Whey and caseins may be included as fillers and binders in nondairy products.

7. You must become a label reader.

IS ANYBODY LISTENING?

I sometimes feel like a "Who" from the book *Horton and the Whos*. I am screaming in the jungle, and no one is listening. I have spent time writing a letter to the founder of a major cancer awareness and support group. I received no response. I talked with the secretary to the educational director of this organization, who told me that her boss would call me "if she was interested." I responded by asking, "How could you not be interested?" I never heard back from her. I was not asking for any money, I had told them; I only wanted them to listen.

I have spent many hours writing letters to the editors of magazines in which ads depicting well-known personalities wearing white milk rings around their mouths appear. I asked the editors to pass on the information that I had provided. In these letters, I again asked only to supply these individuals with information. I did not hear from them.

I have written to the director of the National Cancer Institute, who put me in touch with the Director of Epidemiology, who told me that it would be premature to consider dairy as a causal factor in malignant disease. I wrote him back and asked about women with estrogen-receptor-positive breast cancer. He did not answer my letter. I wrote to the director of the School of Public Health at Harvard and asked him the same question. He did not answer me.

I sent a copy of my book and other supporting information to the director of Health and Human Services. She wrote me back and directed me to a nurse in the National Cancer Institute. I went to a conference in Washington, D.C., that was being held to discuss the African-American disparity in prostate cancer in the U.S. I spoke my piece. They talked about zinc research. I went to the opening of a new cancer prevention research center at a major medical university on open microphone night. I thought they were going to take the microphone out of my hand. The experts would not address my questions appropriately. I have had interest from friends in local African-American churches and have spoken to their congregations. They became even more interested. I received more invitations to speak to their church members. I have sent books to almost all of the members of the Congressional African-American Caucus. I have received no response.

I have not stopped my "cancer from dairy" awareness campaign. I have kept screaming, and people have started to listen. This chapter is about their story.

My message is very clear: You must stop eating dairy products if you want to prevent breast and prostate cancer. Although we have developing evidence of how certain gene defects or mutations cause specific cancers, I do not believe that there could be more clear evidence of how the IGF-1/estrogen combination leads to prostate and probably premenopausal breast cancer. The old adage "you are what you eat" has never been proven to be more accurate, regarding cancer prevention. Can the converse be true? In other words, if you stop what you are eating, can you reverse such cancers as breast and prostate?

Although this book is about prostate cancer, I must relate some information to you that has convinced me that you can, through diet, manipulate certain disease states, including early cancers.

I was about to enter an examining room in one of my satellite offices one morning approximately two years ago when the following encounter occurred. It was the middle of a busy week, and I was a little on the low energy side. One of my nurses noted my lower than normal energy state and said to me, "When you go in that room, it is going to make your day." I entered the room, and one of my female patients of many years blurted out, "Dr. Bibb, thank you for saving my life."

I knew that I had never taken a mole of concern off her, so I was perplexed. She began to tell me that she suffered from fibrocystic disease of the breast. She had suffered from frequent cysts in the breasts, which usually resolved without a problem. A recent episode of her disease resulted in a lump that did not disappear, and a mammogram suggested that the lump was suspicious for cancer. She went through many anxious days until the lump was removed and found to be benign. She related that over a year prior to seeing me for this visit, I had discussed my concerns about dairy consumption being the cause of breast and prostate cancer. She stopped all dairy consumption after her scare, and for the first time in over twenty years, she has not had cysts in her breast associated with her periods. She further related that she had told a friend in California, who also suffered from fibrocystic disease, about her experience. This friend also discontinued dairy and experienced a remission of her fibrocystic disease. I am now aware of twelve women who have had similar experiences.

Fibrocystic disease of the breast is not cancer of the breast, nor is there evidence that this disease results in a higher incidence of breast cancer in the women who suffer from it. These cysts do make it difficult to perform breast self-exams, and even mammograms may not be able to distinguish between benign cysts and malignant tumors. The important point is that certain elements in dairy promote this disease.

Dr. William Danby's work has shown that dairy promotes acne. When I see an acne patient in my office, the first information I provide them is on how consumption of dairy products may aggravate their acne. I have definitely seen how avoidance helps in the acne treatment regimen. This resolution of acne may be related to the IGF-1 in dairy products.

I had a very interesting case in March of 2008. This was a thirty-five-year-old woman who had suffered from hidradenitis suppurativa for eighteen years. This is a condition in which a type of sweat gland gets blocked. These glands exist in the armpits, groin, buttocks, and under the breasts. The disease usually starts in puberty and results in persistent draining abscesses in these areas. It is a painful and embarrassing disease. It is difficult to treat and may require long-term antibiotic use.

As usual, I advised my patient to avoid antiperspirants that might contribute to the blockage, advised the use of antibiotic cleansers, and gave her a prescription for antibiotics. I also advised her to completely avoid dairy. The condition was so severe, I advised her to return in six weeks. On her return, she was almost completely clear. She had not filled the prescription and had not switched to the antibiotic cleanser. She had avoided antiperspirants in the armpits, but the disease occurred in the groin and buttocks also. She was now clear everywhere. I now have four out of four patients with a similar response. I know this is only a four-patient study, but I will say to you, I have been in the private practice of dermatology for twenty-five years and have never seen this disease clear so quickly without prescribed treatment.

I have also tried the dairy-free regimen in men with enlarged prostates. Remember earlier in the book I discussed how estrogens were involved in enlarged prostate? I am happy to report that almost all of these men received significant improvement if not total improvement in urinary hesitancy and frequent urination. This is a sign of their prostate glands shrinking.

I will end the stories I have to tell you with a most interesting recent e-mail to me. A patient of mine attended a lecture I had given about dairy dangers. She had breast pain for over twenty years and had seen numerous doctors at numerous medical institutions. None had helped her. After my lecture she stopped all dairy products, and her pain disappeared. To make sure dairy was the problem, she started dairy consumption again. The pain reappeared. She is now off all dairy products. Her sister suffered from the same problem, and she avoided all dairy products with an identical positive outcome.

The point of the above illustrative stories I have just presented is this: these diseases are thought to be hormonally dependent, and avoidance of dairy resulted in a positive change.

And I have now come to the point where I prepare you for some shocking information about dairy avoidance and positive outcomes regarding cancer.

Most of the men who obtained the results you are about to hear about share similar profiles. There were Caucasians in the age range of sixty to eighty years old. They were frequent dairy users, and they all had prostate cancer that was diagnosed by biopsy. None of the men had metastatic cancer. Their Gleason scores ranged from six to eight. Some were advised to have surgery to remove their cancer, and some were in the process of trying to decide what their options were. I advised all of these men to completely avoid dairy, and they were advised to read all the labels on foods to make sure they were not eating foods with whey or casein. Their PSA values started to drop, and eighty percent with Gleason scores of six or less obtained normal PSA values within six months. Several have undergone repeat prostate biopsies that revealed that the cancer had disappeared!

One man asked his urologist how many times he had seen this happen. The reply from this doctor was that he had never seen this before. Most patients were not comfortable sharing their personal biopsy or lab results. One patient encouraged me to share his biopsy result and even his name. I thought it best to show you his pathology reports only. You saw them in an earlier chapter, but I thought that emphasis would be important: so here they are again.

Figure One: Patient prostate biopsy one year before start of a dairy-free diet.

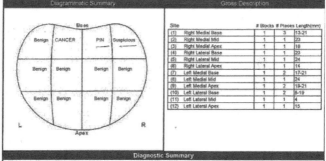

Source: Figure One: Patient's prostate biopsy before dairy avoidance. Reproduced by permission.[2]

Figure Two: Patient biopsy one year after a dairy-free diet.[3]

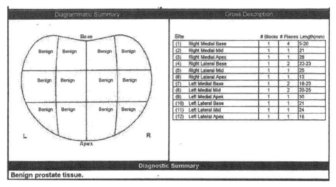

Source: Figure Two: Patient's prostate biopsy one year after diagnosis of prostate cancer and six months after his PSA had returned to normal. Reproduced by permission.[4]

Prostatecancer reversed! Gone! Cured by dietary intervention! And what did I tell my patients to do?

- No intake of obvious dairy products, such as milk, yogurt, cheese, and ice cream.
- No intake of whey-containing products.
- No intake of casein-containing products.

So there you have the answer to whether you can reverse prostate cancer by dietary manipulation. I mentioned earlier that 20 percent of the men with Gleason score six failed to reverse their cancer. The reasons for success and/or failure are not understood at this time.

There are other additional dietary considerations that could increase a man's odds of either reversing or living with prostate cancer. If it does not grow, it does not kill you!

One dietary measure is to consume cooked tomatoes. They contain lycopenes. The tomatoes must be cooked because the lycopenes must be in a certain chemical configuration. Cooking switches them from an inactive form to an active form. If our strategy is to reduce free IGF-1 levels, then lycopenes help you to accomplish this goal because they bind PSA. PSA bound to lycopenes prevents PSA from splitting IGF-1 from its binding protein, effectively lowering levels of free-circulating IGF-1. I try to have marinara sauce at least once a week or eat a six-ounce can of tomato paste weekly. Watermelons are also a good source of lycopenes.

Consume red and/or black raspberries as whole fruit through a blender or as a convenient, raspberry-seed tablet product. Since most of the effective chemical is in the seeds it makes sense to take raspberry-seed tablets. Raspberries contain proven cancer-fighting agents known as *ellagitannins.* Ellagitannins are converted into ellagic acid in our cells, and it is thought that this compound is responsible for the cancer-fighting action of raspberries. Raspberries have at least 220 additional antioxidants that may offer other benefits. I have been involved in this research and have developed a raspberry-seed tablet known as Nixon-Bibb formula®.

Drinking pomegranate juice may offer additional benefit in slowing or preventing prostate cancer. The value of pomegranate consumption has been demonstrated in the lab, and the present theory may be that the high levels of ellagitannins in pomegranate juice may offer benefit through absorption and conversion to ellagic acid.[5]

Try to consume less beef. From our previous chapters on IGF-1 and estrogens, we learned that beef does have low levels of these hormones and protein hormones. We also noted that estrogens survive cooking and that IGF-1 may survive, depending on the cooking temperature.

The consumption of whole soy products, such as tempe, tofu, and soy Silk milk and their effect on prostate cancer have shown varied results with the best effect likely to be prevention as opposed to actual treatment of prostate cancer. Whole soy does contain phyto-estrogens that could stimulate estrogen receptor beta, which theoretically could downregulate prostate cancer.

☠

Most of the beneficial compounds are in whole soy. Soy powders in which the oil has been extracted should be avoided. Soy should be avoided if you have thyroid problems, are taking thyroid medications, and if you have certain types of breast cancer or are on estrogen receptor blocking agents such as Tamoxifen® or Femara®. Seek the advice of your doctor when considering soy consumption if you have cancer. For body builders wishing to avoid isolated soy protein, see Appendix F.

You should eat a lot of broccoli, which can cause certain enzymes (CYP1A1) to be increased. Remember CYP1A1 makes "good" daughter estrogens.

The saying that to help prevent cancer or to modify the course of cancer requires eating a lot of vegetables is definitely true. Eat five to seven helpings of fresh fruit or vegetables daily. This consumption will always serve you well when it comes to preventing prostate cancer and breast cancer.

What You Should Have Learned From This Chapter:

1. Early prostate cancer may be reversible by absolute avoidance of dairy and dairy-related products.

2. Consumption of lycopenes may help reduce blood levels of free IGF-1 by binding PSA.

3. Consumption of raspberries and raspberry-seed products may help fight prostate cancer.

4. Consumption of pomegranate juice may help fight prostate cancer.

5. Consumption of beef and beef products should be reduced or eliminated when combating prostate cancer.

6. Whole soy products may be more useful for prevention of prostate cancer but possibly could help in treatment.

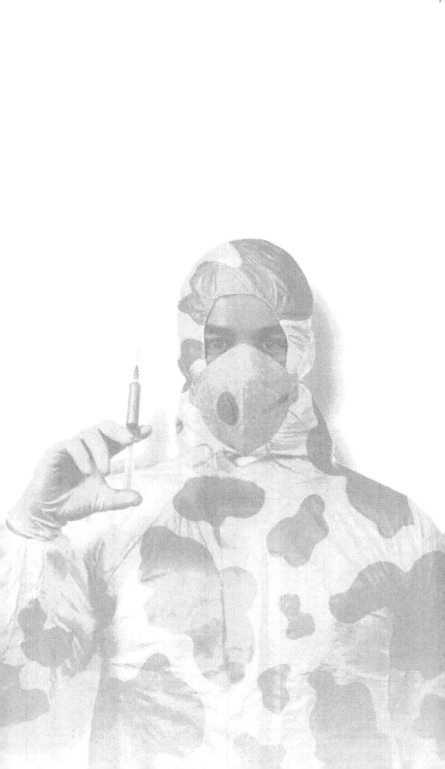

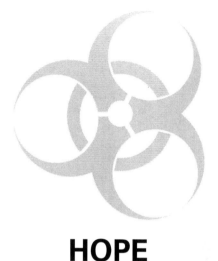

HOPE

In an ABC news article by Associated Press writer Marilynn Marchione, on February 13, 2008, she reports on a recent study of 9,000 older men with prostate cancer. The study was led by Chief Investigator Grace Lu-Yao of the Cancer Institute of New Jersey. These older men had been followed for ten years. The study revealed that in men with low- or moderate-grade tumors, only 3 to 7 percent of them had died of their cancer after ten years.

This study would appear to confirm the "wait and see" option for men in their seventies and eighties diagnosed with early-grade prostate cancer. The article went on to reveal that prostate cancer is the second leading cause of death after lung cancer. Prostatecancer will be diagnosed in 218,000 men in 2008, and globally, 782,000 men will be afflicted with this disease. It is estimated that 254,000 men will die from this killer worldwide.[2]

The "wait and see" option for prostate cancer may be appropriate for older men with prostate cancer but would not be appropriate for younger men, because with years left to live, an aggressive and potentially fatal cancer could develop. This is because as a malignant cell divides, its ability for self-repair is diminished and it, in essence, becomes "more malignant." This may occur because irreversible mutations have occurred in the DNA.

I talked about epimutations in an earlier chapter. These epimutational events have not yet affected permanent changes in the DNA and are reversible. This may be the phenomenon that occurs when dairy is removed from the diet in early prostate cancer and the tumor disappears. Epimutations are the events that result in sections of the p53 gene and other suppressor genes being "turned off." In a turned-off situation, the p53 gene cannot perform its job, that is, to cause death of malignant cells. The message in all this is: keep your p53 gene and other suppressor genes healthy by avoiding dairy.

We also learned that the true incidence of early prostate cancer in younger men may be much higher than is appreciated. The autopsy studies, which we discussed earlier, revealed that 18 percent, 31 percent, and 69 percent of African-American men in their fourth, fifth, and sixth decade of life respectively had early lesions of prostate cancer. The corresponding percentages of Caucasian men were 14 percent, 21 percent, and 38 percent respectively.[3]

It must also be appreciated that a diet of dairy in the newborn or young infant may imprint the animal to have a greater chance of developing prostate or breast cancer later in life. If this process holds true for humans, then the complete avoidance of dairy early in life is an important decision that should be made. One could argue that if we can potentially eliminate prostate cancer in its early stages by dietary elimination of dairy, then why not wait until the diagnosis is made and then become a nondairy user? The problem is that there is a certain failure rate in reversing early prostate cancer with dietary changes alone. Dairy consumption has also been associated with a higher risk of other cancers. It would seem that the most prudent course of action would be to avoid dairy completely.

The cost to treat cancer in the U.S. for 2005 has been estimated at approximately 209.9 billion dollars.[4]

> This includes 74 billion dollars for direct medical costs, 17.5 billion dollars for lost worker productivity due to illness and 118 billion dollars for lost worker productivity due to premature death, both of which are indirect medical costs.[5]

The total direct costs for prostate and breast cancer are estimated at 16.1 billion per year. If indirect costs are proportioned, then these costs for breast and prostate cancer are approximately 29.5 billion per year. This would bring the total costs of prostate and breast cancer to approximately 45.6 billion dollars per year.[6]

Dollar costs cannot measure the emotional pain of having to deal with the diagnosis of cancer. My brother is in the cancer treatment field and has told me about an eighteen-year-old woman with breast cancer that he has treated. In my hometown of Myrtle Beach, South

Carolina, I know of four twenty-year-old women who were given this diagnosis. I also know of a thirty-four-year-old man recently diagnosed with prostate cancer. The horror of having to deal with potential disfigurement or sexual impairment in these early years of age is an angering thought when I know we can substantially prevent or decrease the incidence of these cancers.

The hope lies in the fact that we can take action. I have been involved with other researchers that believe we can make dairy products much safer though the use of certain physical modalities readily available to be put in place. Other additional options exist. During the length of time it takes to put these processes together, we can:

1. Stop impregnating cows shortly after calving. This can reduce the levels of estrogen, PSA, and IGF-1 in their milk.

2. Stop the use of recombinant bovine growth hormones now. This will reduce estrogens and IGF-1 in milk.

3. Stop the use of estrogens in dairy herds now. This can reduce estrogens in their milk.

I must; however, emphasize the fact that cows naturally make estrogens, PSA, and IGF-1, and unless we can eliminate these proteins and hormones in the milk, it will never be completely safe.

What You Should Have Learned From This Chapter:

1. A "wait and see" attitude regarding prostate cancer treatment may not be appropriate for certain older men.

2. A dairy diet at a young age may imprint a person to have a greater risk of prostate cancer later in life.

3. The cost to treat breast and prostate cancer annually may approach fifty billion dollars per year.

4. There is likely a method(s) to make dairy much safer using techniques readily available.

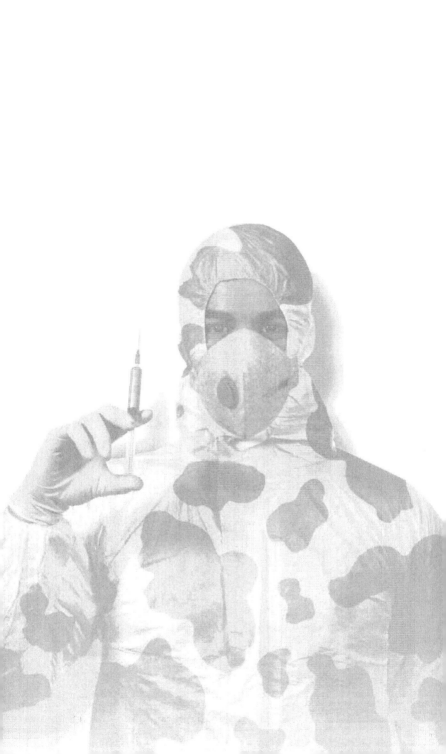

EPILOGUE

An Epidemic

I recently learned of a teenage girl of thirteen with breast cancer. She lives in my community. My brother has treated an eighteen-year-old woman with breast cancer in our state capital. A surgeon friend of mine told me of an eleven-year-old in another state with breast cancer. I mentioned earlier that a breast cancer surgeon in my community has treated at least four women in their early twenties with breast cancer. I know of an eighteen-year-old man with prostate cancer.

If you don't think we are in the midst of an epidemic of breast and prostate cancer, then I guess I must be living on a different planet.

My father died at an early age of non-Hodgkin's lymphoma and his mother at an early age of ovarian cancer.

I mentioned in the earlier portion of this book that I was wrong about the fact that these two cancers were not connected. Let me connect them for you now.

In a Swedish study reported in 2005, Hemminki and Chen reported on 170,000 cancer patients and found that sons had a 1.78 increased risk of developing prostate cancer when their mothers were diagnosed with breast and/or ovarian cancers and 1.39 the risk when their siblings were diagnosed with Hodgkin's lymphoma and/or leukemia.[1]

In a seminal paper in 2006, Pastural and fellow collaborators reported on a suppressor gene known as *RIZ*1. Remember that suppressor genes prevent cancer. This gene was reported as important in preventing the development of chronic-myelogenous leukemia. The authors further stated that this gene was downregulated (turned off) and was associated with the insulin-like growth factor signaling pathway (IGF-1).[2] What this author is saying is that IFG-1 is involved in turning off this important gene, *RIZ*1. Remember that IGF-1 is one of the components of concern in dairy products and further remember that leukemia and prostate cancer are linked by the epidemiologic plots of Dr. William Harris.[3] I think you can see where I am going with this. IGF-1 has been linked to turn off a gene that is important in preventing leukemia.[4] Hodgkin's lymphoma, leukemia, ovarian cancer, breast, and prostate cancer are linked not only through family history of cancer but by Dr. William Harris's analysis of cancer incidence and dairy consumption (see Appendix D).[5] I do not believe that my grandmother's death due to ovarian cancer and my father's death to non-Hodgkin's lymphoma are coincidental. Look at the potential linkage in Table One.

Table One: Genetic linkage events in prostate cancer

EVENT	EFFECT
Mother with ovarian and/or breast cancer	Sons with 1.78 greater risk of developing prostate cancer
Sibling with Hodgkin's lymphoma and/or leukemia	Brothers with 1.39 greater risk of developing prostate cancer
IGF-1 stimulation of IGF-1 receptors in precursor to leukemia cells	Hypermethylation (turn-off) of key suppressor gene known as RIZ1 associated with leukemia
IGF-1 receptor stimulation in prostate cells	Association with increased risk of prostate cancer through hypermethylation of key suppressor genes
Prostate cancer, leukemia, non-Hodgkin's lymphoma, ovarian cancer linked?	Possible genetic linkage of these cancers through hypermethylation (turn-off) of identical key suppressor genes ???

The associational events between cancers that appear to be linked has been explored extensively and reported in a researched, peer-reviewed paper by David S. Shames and colleagues entitled: *"A Genome-Wide Screen for Promoter Methylation in Lung Cancer Identifies Novel Methylation Markers for Multiple Malignancies."*[6] The results of their study regarding common suppressor genes that have been turned off in certain cancers are presented in Table Two.

Table Two: Cancers and their respective methylated genes versus benign tissue methylation of these genes.[7]

Diagnosis	LOX Count	%	MSX1 Count	%	BNC1 Count	%	CTSZ Count	%	ALDH1A3 Count	%	CCNA1 Count	%	NRCAM Count	%	SOX15 Count	%
Breast tumor[a]	16/23	70%	21/23	91%	19/23	83%	14/23	61%	17/23	74%	12/23	52%	4/23	17%	23/23	100%
Lung tumor	**19/20**	**95%**	**11/20**	**55%**	**18/20**	**90%**	**10/20**	**50%**	**9/20**	**45%**	**14/20**	**70%**	**18/20**	**90%**	17/20	85%
Lung benign	4/20	20%	3/20	15%	3/20	15%	0/20	0%	3/20	15%	7/20	35%	8/20	40%	15/20	75%
Breast tumor[b]	**5/14**	**36%**	**11/14**	**79%**	**9/14**	**64%**	**6/14**	**43%**	**4/14**	**29%**	**6/14**	**43%**	ND	ND	**11/14**	**79%**
Breast benign[b]	0/14[c]	0%	5/14	35%	0/14	0%	0/14	0%	0/14	0%	1/14	7%	ND	ND	8/14	57%
Prostate tumor	0/24	0%	**20/24**	**83%**	**18/24**	**75%**	0/24	0%	5/24	21%	**19/24**	**79%**	3/24	13%	24/24	100%
Prostate benign	0/24	0%	10/24	42%	9/24	38%	0/24	0%	7/24	29%	6/24	25%	1/24	4%	21/24	88%
Colon tumor	0/24	0%	**21/24**	**88%**	**22/24**	**92%**	0/24	0%	11/24	46%	24/24	100%	7/24	29%	24/24	100%
Colon benign	0/24	0%	13/24	54%	10/24	42%	0/24	0%	7/17	29%	23/24	96%	4/24	17%	20/24	83%

Numbers in bold face indicate a statistically significant difference in methylation frequency between tumor and normal samples according to a χ^2 statistic ($p < 0.05$). Tissue procurement procedures and clinical information for samples may be found in the Methods section. In brief, all prostate and colon tumors were stage II or later, lung tumors ranged from stage I to IIIB. For breast tumors, see footnotes, below. Benign tissue was obtained from the same patient in all cases except for the UNC samples; see footnotes, below, and Methods.

[a]Breast tumor samples were obtained through a collaboration with Chuck Perou at UNC. Samples in this group were all stage IIB or higher, with the exception of a single stage I tumor.

[b]Breast tumor samples were obtained through a collaboration with David Euhus at UT Southwestern Medical Center. All samples in this group were stage IIB or lower.

[c]Benign breast samples were obtained from the ipsilateral breast except for one sample for LOX and BNC1 and two samples for MSX1, which were obtained from the contralateral breast in the same patient.

doi:10.1371/journal.pmed.0030486.t006

Source: Figure Thirty-Two: Shames D. et al. "A Genome-Wide Screen for Promoter Methylation in Lung Cancer identifies Novel Methylation Markers for Multiple Malignancies," *PLoS Med.* 12 (2006):486. http://www.ncbi.nlm.nih.gov/pmc/articles/PMC1716188/. (In the horizontal lettering are listed the names of the respective suppressor genes, and in the vertical column are the names of the cancers in which the suppressor genes were identified.)

It is not as important that you digest the contents of the chart developed by Shames as it is that you understand what the authors are showing us. They are showing us that certain common suppressor genes are being turned off in the cancers listed in the chart. In other words, it is likely that some common process may be precipitating these cancers by turning off the suppressor genes that prevent a person from getting these cancers.

This sounds like a science-fiction novel. Some common dietary practice in Western societies may be turning off our protective genes, likely resulting in teenagers with breast cancer and African-American men with incipient prostate cancer in their thirties and forties. And, more importantly, we may also be passing these turned off genes on to the next generation.

I was discussing my book with my son Jon recently. He was relating to me how odd it seems that people are likely walking around, thinking to themselves that prostate cancer and breast cancer are unavoidable. It is just a fact of life they must think, he pondered.

Jon's thoughts reminded me of a true story that I read about a number of years ago.

A number of cows were lined up single file, as they were penned in by fences on either side. They were headed into a slaughterhouse. One particular cow decided to jump the fence and run. He came to a river and swam across it, eluding his pursuers. He wandered around for several days before he was caught. The farmer who owned the cow decided to let him live out his days. He thought that the cow should have this option, since he was determined to live.

And so it seems with humans. We wait in line for our cancers to develop, not realizing that the very food we were taught was good for us is, in fact, killing us.

Do not accept these cancers as a fact of life. Be determined to swim across the river.

GLOSSARY

ACTH: Adrenocorticotropin hormone. It is a major hormone that stimulates the adrenal gland to release other hormones and hormone precursors. It is released from the pituitary gland and circulates through the bloodstream as an endocrine hormone stimulating such compounds as androstenedione and DHEA and DHEA sulfate to be released from the adrenal gland.

Adrenal gland: This is a gland that sits up top of each kidney. It is responsible for releasing hormones that can be converted into male hormones in the prostate gland. It is stimulated to release hormones by ACTH.

Age adjusted: This means that a population being studied has been adjusted using a weighted average using a specific population for which the comparisons are made. Age adjustment for the U.S. statistical base uses these averages based on the U.S population in the year 2000. An age adjustment means that the cancer statistics you look at are not caused by an aging population.

Apoptosis: This is defined as natural cell death in which the cell absorbs and recycles its contents for reuse. The biochemistry of the cell normally uses this process to cause cells to die that have been injured beyond repair or have become malignant.

Autocrine: Usually refers to a cell producing a hormone or protein that, in turn, binds and affects the cell type that produced it.

Binding protein: A protein that binds to its cofactor hormone or protein. Typically in the systems we look at in this book, it would be a factor that diminishes the biologic activity of a particular hormone.

Bladder: The biologic storage vessel for urine. Below it sits the prostate gland. When the prostate gland enlarges, it can restrict the flow of urine from the bladder.

Case-controlled study: This type of study is used to see if a particular disease has an association with some environmental factor. People with a particular disease or problem are chosen; then, retrospectively, an attempt is made to associate the disease with the environmental factor, such as diet. An example would be to choose men of a particular age with prostate cancer and then question them about diet to see if an association can be made.

C2: One of the "good" daughter estrogens produced by CYP1A1. C2 is synonymous with 2-hydroxyestrone. It preferentially stimulates estrogen receptor beta, which would help prevent cancer of the breast or prostate.

C16: One of the "bad" daughter estrogens known as 16 alpha-hydroxyestrone produced by the enzyme CYP1B1. It preferentially stimulates estrogen receptor alpha, which would help promote cancer of the breast or prostate.

Casein: The solid portion of milk that is created when the fat-soluble proteins of milk are precipitated out of milk during the cheese-making process. Most casein is used to make cheese. Casein can also be used as a binding agent in certain foods.

Cohort study: This is a longitudinal study over time in which two similar groups are compared as to the outcome of a treatment or exposure being studied. For example, one group consuming dairy products could be compared to another group not consuming dairy products over time, and then the incidence of prostate cancer could be compared in each group.

CpG island: A group of coupled cytosine-guanine complexes that can control the expression of a gene. When these couplets become attached to methyl groups and the entire complex receives methyl group attachment, the gene can be considered "turned off." They should be considered as the switches used to turn a gene on or off.

CYP1A1: An enzyme that can convert naturally occurring estrogens, such as estrone into "good" daughter estrogens, such as 2-hydroxyestrone (C2).

CYP1B1: An enzyme that can convert naturally occurring estrogens into "bad" daughter estrogens, such as 16 alpha-hydroxyestrogen (C16).

Cytosine: A chemical known as a pyrimidine base. It is one of the constituents of DNA.

DNA: Deoxyribonucleic acid. This is the so-called double helix, which contains all the genes that control us as human beings.

Denature: To render inactive. In biological systems it generally implies that a protein has been rendered biologically inactive.

Differentiation: The development of a specialized type of cell from a less specialized cell. In terms of cancer, differentiation means how differently the cancer compares to the normal parent cell.

Disulfide bonds: The linkage of two sulfur atoms. Disulfide links are typically used by proteins to maintain their biologically active configurations.

Epigenetic: The process by which the function of a gene is modified through a process other than a permanent mutation in a gene. This can be accomplished by attaching methyl groups to CpG islands, rendering a gene "turned off." The process is also used to turn genes "on."

Epithelial cells: The cells that line the skin and organs.

Endogenous: Occurring within the body.

Ergosterol: A steroid-like compound occurring in plants. It can be a precursor compound to vitamin D.

Estrogens: Female hormones. They include estrone, estradiol, and estratriol. The most potent estrogen is 17 beta estradiol.

Estrogen receptor: Receivers of estrogen located on or in cells. Breast and prostate tissue, as well as other hormonally sensitive tissues, have these receptors. The main receptors of estrogen on prostate and breast cells are called alpha and beta. Generally if an estrogen compound attaches to an alpha receptor, a cell could progress toward malignancy. If an estrogen compound attaches to a beta receptor, then a cell would be protected from becoming malignant.

Estrogenic: Behaving like an estrogen. Compounds are tested in the lab for their ability to make cancerous breast tissue grow. If growth occurs, then the compound is said to be estrogenic.

Exogenous: Outside the body.

Guanine: A chemical known as a purine base. It is one of the constituents of DNA.

Gleason score: This is a score total given to the pathologic examination of prostate tissue, using a grading score of most differentiated to least differentiated with a grading system of 1–5, with 1 being the most differentiated (like a normal cell). It is the sum of the most common cell type grade added to the grade of the second most common cell type. A grade of two is the lowest score, with 10 being the highest score. The higher scores generally correlate with poorer prognoses.

Heat map: This is a map correlating the degree of methylation of a gene ("turned off") with the color red. Red indicates fully "turned off" genes with white meaning fully "turned on." The subsequent maps of the major suppressor genes investigated look like the burning coals of a fire. This is an investigational tool that can compare different cancers with the major suppressor genes that are hypermethylated (turned off).

Hormone: A chemical compound produced by a cell that is carried in the bloodstream and targets another cell causing an end result. An example would be ACTH, which is released by the pituitary gland and targets the adrenal gland to release other hormones.

Hypothalamus: A part of the brain that can cause the pituitary gland to release hormones, including leutinizing hormone. Leutinizing hormone causes the testis to release testosterone.

IGF-1: Insulin-like-growth factor one. This is a protein produced naturally in the liver of humans but is also secreted in the milk of cows. IGF-1 produces the effects of growth hormone, which is to cause cells to grow. The IGF-1 produced by cows is identical to human insulin-like growth factor one.

Incidence: The frequency at which a particular disease or problem occurs in a population.

Leutinizing hormone: A hormone released from the pituitary gland that stimulates the testis to release testosterone.

Meiosis: The process in which sperm and eggs are created. The chromosome number is reduced to one half that of an adult cell.

Methylation: The process of attaching a methyl ($CH3$) group to CpG couplets in a suppressor gene, in effect, turning it off.

Microgram: One millionth of a gram.

Milligram: One-thousandth of a gram.

Mitosis: The process of a mother cell dividing into two identical cells.

Nanogram: One-billionth of a gram.

Necrosis: Cell death characterized by the release of the cellular content, damaging adjacent cells.

Needle biopsy: A process in which tissue is obtained by guiding a needle into the tissue of interest and obtaining a tissue specimen. It would be used to obtain a specimen without an open operative procedure. This procedure is used to obtain biopsy specimens of the prostate gland when cancer is suspected.

Oncogene: A gene that allows cells to become immortal, transitioning them into cancer. An example is the bcl 2 gene.

Ovary: The female organ that produces eggs.

Paracrine: The process in which a cell produces a hormone or protein that influences or affects adjacent cells.

P53 gene: A major suppressor gene. This gene controls apoptosis, or programmed cell death. When a cell becomes defective or malignant, this gene will normally cause the cell to die. This gene has been found to be defective in approximately 50 percent of human cancers.

Phytoestrogen: A plant-based, estrogen like chemical. Some plant-based phyto-estrogens have shown benefit in cancer prevention or treatment.

Picogram: One-billionth of a gram.

PIN: Prostate intraepithelial neoplasia. The earliest change in prostate cells leading to the development of prostate cancer.

Protein: A combination of amino acids. It is produced through the genetic codes contained in genes.

PSA: Prostate-specific antigen. It is a sugar-linked protein, which is produced by both normal and malignant prostate cells. It can be useful in determining the possibility that a man might have prostate cancer. It plays an active role in prostate cancer by splitting IGF-1 from its binding protein.

P-value: A mathematical term used to describe how precisely two values may be related in a linear fashion. The smaller the p-value, the closer the association.

Quinone: A highly reactive derivative estrogen chemical that can cause mutations in genes. Quinone compounds are thought to play a role in the development of breast and prostate cancer.

Rachitis: A term that describes the effect of vitamin D deficiency on the bones.

Rickets: The deficiency of vitamin D.

Regression analysis: A mathematical technique to determine if the relationship between two variables can be described by a straight line.

SEER: Surveillance Epidemiology and End Results. The U.S. government's statistical database for disease processes.

Seminal fluid: The fluid in which is carried the sperm.

Suppressor gene: A gene that helps prevent cancer. There have been a number of them described to date. Cancer is caused by the shutdown of suppressor genes.

Whey: The liquid portion of milk left over from the cheese-making process. It contains IGF-1 and water-soluble estrogens.

ENDNOTES

Prostate Cancer: The Disease

1 Wikipedia, "Reproductive System", http://en.wikipedia.org/wiki/Reproductive_system. (accessed Nov. 14, 2009).

2 Ibid.

3 Dreamstime, "Prostatic tissue young human," http://www.dreamstime.com/royalty-free-stock-photos-prostatic-tissue-young-human-image6166778. (accessed Nov.7, 2009), Reproduced by licensure.

4 Ibid.

5 Ibid.

6   Fernández, PL, et al., "Alterations of cell cycle-regulatory genes in prostate cancer." Pathobiology 701 (2002): 1–10.

7   U.S. Dept of Health and Human Services. National Cancer Institute, Normal Cell Division.png, http://press2.nci.nih.gov/sciencebehind/cancer/cancer01.htm. (accessed Nov 7, 2009).

8   U.S. Dept of Health and Human Services. National Cancer Institute, Normal Cell Division.png, http://press2.nci.nih.gov/sciencebehind/cancer/cancer01.htm. (accessed Nov. 7, 2009).

Cancer Cell Division.png, http://press2.nci.nih.gov/sciencebehind/cancer/cancer01.htm.(accessed Nov 7, 2009).

10   Ibid.

11   Kellokumpu-Lehtinen, P, et al., "Leukemia-inhibitory factor stimulates breast, kidney and prostate cell proliferation by paracrine and autocrine pathways." Intl Nat. J Cancer 66 (1996): 515–19.

12   Daniel O'Sullivan., Endocrine Effects on the Prostate Gland. (2008) Reproduced by permission.

13   Daniel O'Sullivan., Paracrine Stimulation. (2008) Reproduced by permission.

14 Daniel O'Sullivan., Autocrine Stimulation. (2008) Reproduced by permission.

15 Patient H.W., abnormal prostate biopsy prior to dairy-free diet., copy of biopsy report given to author by patient. (2008) Reproduced by permission.

16 Ibid.

17 Patient H.W., normal prostate biopsy after one year on a dairy-free diet, copy of biopsy report given to author by patient. (2008) Reproduced by permission.

18 Ibid.

19 Wikipedia, "Gleason Staging System, Gleason Score", http://en.wikipedia. org/wiki/Gleason_staging_system. (accessed Nov.7, 2009).

Prostate Cancer: The Statistics

1   American Cancer Society, "Cancer Facts & Figures", http://www.cancer.org/ downloads/STT/caFF2006PWSecured. pdf(accessed N0v 7, 2009).

2   Peter Montague, "HEADLINES: CANCER TRENDS," *Rachel's Environment and Health Weekly* ,550, 12, June 1997, *http://www. re-action.com/dc/news/rachels/rach*1550. *html(accessed* June 15 2008).

3   Yatani, R., "Trends in Frequency of Latent Prostate Cancer In Japan from 1965–1979 To 1982–1986,". *J Natl Cancer Instit.* 80 (1988): 683–7.

4   Sakr, WA., "*Epidemiology of high grade prostatic intraepithelial Neoplsia,*" *Pathol Res Pract* 80 (1995): 883–7.

5   Sánchez, CM., "Prevalence Of Prostatic Intraepithelial Neoplasia in Spain," *Arch Esp Ur* 01.54 (2001): 11039.

6   Soos, G., et al., "The Prevalence Of Prostate Carcinoma and Its Precursor in Hungary: an Autopsy Study," *Eur Urol* 48 (2005): 739–44.

7   Dewailly, E., et al., "Inuit are Protected Against Prostate Cancer," *Cancer Epidemiol Biomarkers Prev* 12 (2003): 926–7.

8   Ibid.

9   MacLean, CH., et al., "Effects of Omega-Fatty Acid On Cancer Risk: A Systematic Review," *JAMA* 295 (2006): 403–15.

Food Association Studies

1   Talamini, R., et al.,"Nutrition, Social Factors and Prostatic Cancer in a Northern Italian Population," Br J Cancer 53 (1986): 817–21.

2   Mettlin, C., et al., "Beta-"Carotene and Animal Fats and Their Relationship to Prostate Cancer Risk. A Case Controlled Study," Cancer 64 (1989): 605–12.

3   LaVecchia, C., et al., "DairyProducts
    and the Risk of Prostatic Cancer,"
    Oncology 48 (1991): 406–10.

4   Chan, JM., et al., "DairyProducts,
    Calcium, Phosphorous, Vitamim D
    and Risk of Prostate Cancer (Sweden),"
    Cancer Causes Control 9 (1998): 559–66.

5   Grant, WB., "An Ecologic Study of
    Dietary Links to Prostate Cancer,"
    Altern Med Rev 4 (1999): 162–9.

6   Bosetti, C., et al., "Fraction of
    Prostate Cancer Incidence Attributed
    to Diet in Athens, Greece," Eur J
    Cancer Prev 9 (2000): 119–23.

7   Chan, JM., et al., "Dairy Products,
    Calcium, and Prostate Cancer Risk
    in the Physicians' Health Study," Am
    J Clin Nutr 74 (2001): 549–54.

8   Ibid.

9   Qin, LQ., et al., "Milk Consumption is
    a risk factor for prostate cancer: meta-
    analysis of case controlled Studies,"
    Nutr Cancer 48 (2004): 22–7.

10 Bosetti, C., et al.,"Food Groups and
    Risk of Prostate Cancer in Italy,"
    Int J Cancer 110 (2004): 424–8.

11 Keese, E., et al.,"Dairy Products, Calcium and Phosphorous Intake, and the Risk Of Prostate Cancer: Results of the French Prospective SU.VI.MAX (Supplémentation en Vitamines et Minéraux Antioxydants) Study," Br J Nutr 95 (2006): 539–45.

12 Rohrmann, S., et al.,"Meat And Dairy Consumption And Subsequent Risk Of Prostate Cancer in a US Cohort Study," Cancer Causes Control 18 (2007): 41–50.

13 Mitrou, PN., et al., "A prospective study of dietary calcium, dairy products and prostate cancer risk (Finland),"Int J Cancer 120 (2007): 2466–73.

14 Kurahashi, N., et al.,"DairyProduct, Saturated Fatty Acid, and CalciumIntakeand ProstateCancer in a Prospective Cohort of Japanese Men," Cancer Epidemiol Biomarkers Prev 17 (2008): 930–7.

15 Ibid.

16 Ibid.

17 Harris, W M.D., "Cancer and the Vegetarian Diet," (1999), http://www.vegsource.com/harris/cancer_vegdiet.htm (accessed Feb. 8, 2008).

18 Ibid.

19 Ibid.

20 Ibid.

Harry Steenbock and the Antirachitic Machine

1 Schneider, H., "Harry Steenbock (1886–1967)," Journal of Nutrition, http://jn.nutrition.org/cgi/reprint/103/9/1233.pdf (accessed Nov 3, 2009).

2 Ibid.

3 Robert D. Bibb, M.D., Conversion of ergosterol to vitamin D2 by ultraviolet light. Reproduced by permission.

4 Ibid.

5 Steenbock, H., United States Patent and Trademark Office, Patent Number 1,680,818 "Antirachitic Products and Process," issued to Dr. Harry Steenbock 1928, http://www.strategicpatentlaw.com/ (accessed June 15, 2008).

6 Satin, M., American Council on Science and Health, (2003) "Pasteurization and Irradiation," http://foodhaccp.com/msgboard.mv?parm_func+showmsg+parm_msgnum+1010717 (accessed Nov. 7, 2009).

7 Schneider, H., "Harry Steenbock (1886–1967)" Journal of Nutrition, http://jn.nutrition.org/cgi/reprint/103/9/1233.pdf (accessed Nov 3 2009).

8 Ibid.

9   Wkipedia ,"Harry Steenbock
    in his laboratory, 1923,",http://
    en.wikipedia.org/wiki/Harry_
    Steenbock (accessed Nov 7, 2009).

10 Steenbock, H., United States Patent
    and Trademark Office, Patent Number
    1,680,818 "Antirachitic Products and
    Process," issued to Dr. Harry Steenbock
    1928, http://www.strategicpatentlaw.
    com/ (accessed June 15, 2008).

11 Ibid.

12 Grosvenor, CE., et al., "Hormones
    and Growth Factors in Milk,"
    EndocrineReviews 14 (1992): 710–727.

13 Daniel O'Sullivan, Folded Protein
    (2008). Reproduced by permission.

14 Daniel O'Sullivan. Ultraviolet
    light denaturing a protein (2008).
    Reproduced by permission.

15 Daniel O'Sullivan. Folded Protein
    (2008) Reproduced by permission.

16 Daniel O'Sullivan. Ultraviolet
    light denaturing a protein (2008)
    Reproduced by permission.

17 Ibid.

18 Ibid.

19 Dr. Lyndom Larcom, e-mail message
    to author, January 6, 2004.

20 Ibid.

Insulin-like Growth Factor One

1   De Jong, F.H., et al., "Peripheral Hormone
    Levels in Controls and Patients with
    Prostate Cancer or BenignProstatic
    Hyperplasia: Results from the Dutch-
    Japanese Case-Control Study," Cancer
    Research 51 (1991): 3445–3450.

2   Grosvenor, C., et al., "Hormones
    and Growth Factors in Milk,"
    EndocrineReviews 14 (1993): 710–28.

3   Shaneyfelt, T., et al., "Hormonal predictors
    of prostate cancer: a meta-analysis," J
    Clinical Oncology 18 (2000): 847–53.

4   Hankinson, SE., et al., "Circulating
    Concentrations of Insulin-Like
    Growth Factor-1 and Risk of Breast
    Cancer," Lancet 351(1998): 1393–6.

5   Tiryakioaylu, O., et al., "Age dependency of
    serum insulin-like growth factor (IGF-1)
    in healthy Turkish adolescents and adults,"
    Ind J Med Sciences 57 (2003): 543–48.

6   Collier, R J., et al., "Factors Affecting
    Insulin-Like Growth Factor-1
    Concentration in Bovine Milk," J
    DairyScience 74 (1991) Sep: 2905–11.

7   Rajaram, S., et al., "Insulin-Like Growth Factor-Binding Proteins in Serum and Other Biological Fluids: Regulation and Functions," Endocrine Reviews 18 (1997): 801–831.

8   Chan, JM., et al., "Plasma Insulin-Like Growth Factor -1 and Prostate Cancer Risk: a Prospective Study," Science 279 (1998): 563–6.

9   Shaneyfelt, T., et al., "Hormonal predictors of prostate cancer: a meta-analysis," Journal of Clinical Oncology 18 (2000): 847–53.

10 Jenkins, PJ., "Cancers Associated with Acromegaly," Neuroendocrinolgy 83(2006): 218–23.

11 Shevah, O., et al., "Patients with congenital deficiency of IGF-1 seem protected from the development of malignancies: a preliminary report," Growth Hormone IGF Res 17 (2007): 54–7.

12 Signorello, LB., et al., "Lifestyle Factors and Insulin-Like Growth-1 Levels Among Elderly Men," Eur J Cancer Pre 9 (2000): 173–8.

13 Majeed, N., et al., "A germ line mutation that delays prostate cancer progression and prolongs survival in a murine prostate cancer model," Oncogene 24 (2005): 4736–40.

14 Stattin, P., et al., "High Levels of Circulating Insulin-Like Growth Factor-1 Increase Prostate Cancer Risk: a Prospective Study in a Population-Based Nonscreened Cohort," J Clinical Oncology 22 (2004): 3104–12.

15 Xu, RJ.,et al., "Gastrointestinal Absorption of Insulin-Like Growth Factor-1 in Neonatal Pigs," J Pediatric Gastrointestinal Nutrition23 (1996): 430–7.

16 Philipps, AF., et al., "Growth of artificially fed infant rats: effect of supplementation with insulin-like growth factor -1," Am J Physiology 272 (1997): 532–9.

17 Kimura, T., et al., "Gastrointestinal Absorption of Recombinant Human Insulin-Like Growth Factor-1 in Rats," J Pharmacol Exp Ther 283 (1997): 611–8.

18 Philipps, AF., et al., "Absorption of milk-borne insulin-like growth factor-1 into portal blood of suckling rats," J Pediatric Gastrointestinal Nutri 31 (2000): 128–35.

19 Cadogan, J., et al., "Milk intake and bone mineral acquisition in adolescent girls: randomized controlled intervention trial," British J of Medicine 315 (1997): 1255–60.

20 Heaney, RP., et al., "Dietary changes favorably affect bone remodeling in older adults," J Am Diet Assoc 9 (1999): 1228–33.

21 Rich-Edwards, JW., et al., "Milk consumption and the prepubertal somatotropic axis," Nutri J 6 (2007): 28.

22 Dennis, Liu, PhD., Howard Hughes Medical Institute, "p53: The Guardian of the Genome,", http://www.hhmi.org/biointeractive/cancer/p53/01.html (accessed 2009).

23 Adams, TE., et al. "Structure and function of the type 1 insulin-like growth factor receptor," Cell Mol Life Sci 57 (2000): 1050–93.

24 Meyers, FJ., et al., "Very frequent p53 mutations in metastatic prostate cancer and in matched primary tumors.", Cancer 12 (1998): 2534–9.

25 Adams, TE., et al., "Structure and function of the type 1 insulin-like growth factor receptor," Cell Mol Life Sci 57 (2000): 1050–93.

26 Ibid.

27 Mendouncesa-Rodriquez, CA., et al., "Tumor suppressor gene P53: mechanisms of action in cell proliferation and death," Rev Invest Clin 53 (2001): 266–73.

28 Meyers, FJ., et al., "Very frequent p53 mutations in metastatic prostate cancer and in matched primary tumors," Cancer 12 (1998): 2534–9.

29 Troester, MA., et al., "Gene expression patterns associated with p53 status in breast cancer," BMC Cancer 6 (2006): 276.

30 Grzmil, M., et al., "Blockade of the type 1 IGF receptor expression in human prostate cancer cells inhibits proliferation and invasion, up regulates IGF-1 binding protein-3 and suppresses MMP-2 expression," J Path 202 (2004): 50–9.

31 Neuberg, M., et al., "The p53/IGF-1 receptor axis in the regulation of programmed Cell death," Endocrine 7 (1997): 107–9.

32 Adams, TE., et al., "Structure and function of the Type 1 insulin-like growth factor receptor," Cell Mol Life Sci 57 (2000): 1050–93.

33 Grosvenor, CE., et al., "Hormones and Growth Factors in Milk," Endocrine Reviews 14 (1992): 710–727.

34 Pandini, G., et al., " 17 Beta-estradiol up-regulates the insulin-like growth factor receptor through a nongenotropic pathway in prostate cancer cells," Cancer Res. 18 (2007): 8932–41.

35 Ibid.

36 Surmacz, E., et al., "Role of estrogen receptor alpha in modulating IGF-1receptor signaling and function in breast cancer," J Exp Clin Cancer Res 23 (2004): 385–94.

37 Dipoala, RS., et al., "Overcoming bcl-2 and p53 resistance in prostate cancer," Semin Oncol 26 (1999): 112–6.

Estrogens

1 Larcom, L. PhD. Personal communication with author, Sept. 2009.

2 Wikipedia,"Estrogen,",http://en.wikipedia.org/wiki/Estrogen(accessed Nov. 7, 2009).

3 Ibid.

4 Ibid.

5 Ibid

6 Ibid.

7 Pattarozzi, A. et al., "17 -Estradiol pormotes breast cancer cell proliferation, inducing SDF-1 mediated EGFR transactivation: reversal by gefitinib pretreatment," Molecular Pharm. 73 (2007): 191–02.

8 Ramagopalan, SV., et al., "Age of puberty and the risk of multiple sclerosis: a population based study," Eur J Neurol. 3 (2009): 342–7.

9 Graham MJ. et al., "Secular trend in age in China: a case study of two rural counties in Anhui Province," J Biosoc Sci 2(1999): 257–67.

10 International Programme on Chemical Safety, World Health Organization 2000, "WHO Food Additives Series: 43,": http://www.inchem.org/documents/jecfa/jecmono/v43jec05.htm (accessed Nov.7, 2009).

11 Henricks, DM., et al., "Residue Levels of Endogenous Estrogens in Beef Tissues," J of Animal Science 57 (1983): 247–255.

12 Wolford, ST., et al., "Measurement of Estrogens in Cow's Milk, Human Milk and Dairy Products," J Dairy Science 62 (1979): 1458–63.

13 Malekinejad H., "Naturally Occurring Estrogens in Processed Milk and in Raw Milk (from Gestated Cows)," J Agric Food Chem 54 (2006): 9785–91.

14 Ibid.

15 Wolford, ST., et al., "Measurement of Estrogens in Cow's Milk, Human Milk and Dairy Products," J Dairy Science 62 (1979): 1458–63.

16 Daxenberger, A., et al., "Possible impact of animal oestrogens in food," Human Reprod. Update 7 (2001): 340–55.

17 Ibid.

18 Anderson, A., et al., "Exposure to exogenous estrogens in food: possible impact on human health development," Eur J of End 0.140 (1999): 477–85.

19 Daxenberger, A., et al., "Possible Impact of Animal Oestrogens in Food," Human Reprod. Update 7 (2001): 340–55

19 García-Peláez B. "Technical Note: Measurement of Total Estrone Content in Foods. Application to Dairy Products," J of Dairy Science 82 (2004): 2331–2336.

20 Serrano-Mu ounces, M., et al., "Intestinal oleoyl-estrone esterase activity in the Wistar Rat," J Endocrinolol Invest 31 (2008): 125–31.

21 Cabot, C., et al., "In the rat, estrone sulphate is the main serum metabolite of oral oleoyl-estrone," J Endocrinol Invest 30 (2007): 376–81.

22 Wikipedia, "File: Testosterone estradiol conversion.png", http://en.wikipedia.org/wiki/File:Testosterone_estradiol_conversio.png (accessed Nov.7, 2009).

23 Henricks, DM., et al., "Residue levels of endogenous estrogens in beef tissues," J of Animal Science 57 (1983): 247–255.

24 Ibid

25 Ibid.

26 Henricks, DM., et al., "Endogenous Estrogens In Bovine Tissues," J of Animal Science 45 (1977): 652–8.

27 Ibid.

28 Dunn, TG., et al., "Metabolites of Estradiol-17 and Estradiol-17-Benzoate in Bovine Tissues," J of Animal Science 45 (1977): 659–73.

29 Schindler, AE., et al., "Comparative pharmacokinetics of oestradiol, oestrone, oestrone sulfate and "conjugated estrogens" after oral administration," Arzneimittelforschung 32 (1982): 787–91.

30 infoplease® Pearson Education 2000–2009 " Per Capita Consumption of Principal Foods,", http://www.infoplease.com/ipa/A0104742.html.

31 Henricks, DM., et al., "Endogenous Estrogens In Bovine Tissues," J of Animal Science 45 (1977): 652–8.

32 García-Peláez, B., et al., "Technical Note: Measurement of Total Estrone Content In Foods. Application to Dairy Products," J of Dairy Science 82 (2004): 2331–2336.

33 U.S. Department of Agricultural Statistics Service ,"Dairy Products 2005 Summary April 2006 Da2–1(06),",http://quickstats.nass.usda.gov/ (accessed Nov.7, 2009).

34 Schultz M. "Dairy Products Profile," (2005), http://www.agmrc.org/agrmc/commodity/livestock/dairy/dairyproductsprofile.htm (accessed Feb. 9, 2008).

35 The Pew Charitable Trusts (2008), http://www.pewtrusts.org//our_work_report_detail.aspx?id+35312 (accessed Nov. 7, 2009).

36 García-Peláez, B., et al., "Technical Note: Measurement of Total Estrone Content in Foods. Application to Dairy Products," J of Dairy Science 82 (2004): 2331–2336.

37 Remesar X. et al., " Estrone in food: a factor influencing the development of obesity?," Eur J Nutr 38 (1999): 247–53.

38 Pape-Zambito, DA., et al., "Concentrations of 17-estradiol in Holstein whole milk," Journal of Dairy Science 90 (2007): 3308–13.

39 Daxenberger, A., et al., "Possible health impact of animal oestrogens in food," Human Reprod Update 7 (2001): 340–55.

40 Li-Quang, Qin, et al.,"Estrogen: one of the risk factors in milk for prostate cancer," Medical Hypotheses 62 (2004): 133–42.

41 Chavarro, JE., et al., "A prospective study of dairy foods intake and anovulatory infertility," Human Reproduction 22 (2007):1340–7.

42 Farlow, D., et al., "Quantitative measurement of endogenous estrogen metabolites, risk-factors for development of breast cancer, in commercial milk products by LC-MS/MS," J Chromatography B Analyt Technol Biomed Life Sci 877(2009): 1327–34.

43 Ganmaa, D., et al., "Commercial cows' milk has uterotrophic activity on the uteri of young ovariectomized rats and immature rats," Int Journal Cancer 118 (2006): 2363–5.

44 Guillemette, C. et al., "Metabolic inactivation of estrogens in breast tissue by UDP-glucuronosyltransferase enzymes: an overview," Breast Cancer Research. 6 (2004): 246–54.

45 Ganmaa, D., et al., "Commercial cows' milk has uterotrophic activity on the uteri of young ovariectomized rats and immature rats," Int Journal Cancer 118 (2006): 2363–5.

46 Larrson, SC. et. al., "Milk and lactose intakes and ovarian cancer risk in the swedish mammography cohort," Am J Clin Nutr 80 (2004):1353–7.

47 Ganmaa, D., et al., "Commercial cows' milk has uterotrophic activity on the uteri of young ovariectomized rats and immature rats," Int Journal Cancer 118 (2006): 2363–5.

48 Carruba, G. "Estrogen and prostate cancer: an eclipsed truth in an androgen dominated scenario," Journal Cell Biocemistry 102 (2007): 899–911.

49 Risbridger, GP. et al., "Estrogen action on the prostate gland: a critical mix of endocrine and paracrine signaling," Journal Of Molecular Endocrinology 39 (2007): 183–8.

50 Larcom, L. PhD. Personal communication with author, Sept. 2009.

51 Risbridger, GP. et al., "Estrogen action on the prostate gland: a critical mix of endocrine and paracrine signaling," Journal Of Molecular Endocrinology 39 (2007): 183–8.

52 Grosvenor, C. et al., "Hormones and growth factors in milk," Endocrine Reviews 14 (1993): 710–28.

53 Lukaczer, D. "Estrogen's Two-Way Street," Nutr Science News Nov. (2001), http://www.newhope.com/ nutritionsciencenews/nsn_backs/Nov_01/ estrogen.cfm (accessed Nov.7, 2009).

54 Ibid.

55 Ibid.

56 Immuna Care Corporation, 2007 "General information,", http://www.estrametimmunacare.com (accessed Jan. 15, 2008).

57 Mingzhou, S., et al., "Cytochrome P4501A1-inhibitory action of antimutagenic anthraquinones in medicinal plants and the structure-activity relationship," Bios,Biotech, and Biochem. 64 (2000): 1373–78.

58 Zhu, BT. et al., "Quantitative structure-activity relationship of various endogenous estrogen metabolites for human estrogen receptor and subtypes: insights into the structural determinants favoring a differential subtype binding," Endocrinology 147 (2006): 4132–50.

59 Risbridger, G., et al., "Estrogen action on the prostate gland: a citical mix of endocrine and paracrine signaling," Journal Of Molecular Endocrinology 39 (2007): 183–188.

60 Risbridger, G., et al., "Estrogen action on the prostate gland: a citical mix of endocrine and paracrine signaling," Journal Of Molecular Endocrinology 39 (2007): 183–188.

61 Zhu, BT. et al., "Quantitative structure-activity relationship of various endogenous estrogen metabolites for human estrogen receptor and subtypes: insights into the structural determinants favoring a differential subtype binding," Endocrinology 147 (2006): 4132–50.

62 Ibid.

63 Ibid.

64 Ibid/

65 Farlow, D., et al., "Quantitative measurement of endogenous estrogen metabolites, risk-factors for development of breast cancer, in commercial milk products by LC-MS/MS," J Chromatography B Analyt Technol Biomed Life Sci 877(2009):1327–34.

66 Dawling, S., et al., "Methoxyestrogens exert feedback inhibition on cytochrome P450 1A1 and 1B1," Cancer Research 15 (2003): 3127–3132.

67 Navas, J., et al., "Estrogen-mediated suppression of cytochrome p4501A(CYP1A1) expression in rainbow trout hepatocytes: role of estrogen receptor," Chem Biol Interact 38 (2001): 285–98.

68 Hanna, I H., et al., "Cytochrome P450 1B1 (CYP1B1) pharmacogenetics: association of polymorphisms with functional

differences in estrogen hydroxylation activity," Cancer Res 60 (2000):3440–4.

69 Yuki, T., et al., "Human CYP1B1 Is Regulated by Estradiol via Estrogen Receptor," Cancer Res 64 (2004):3119–3125.

70 Risbridger, G., et al., "Estrogen action on the prostate gland: a critical mix of endocrine and paracrine signaling," Journal of Molecular Endocrinology 39 (2007):183–188.

71 Ragavan, N., et al., "CYP1B1 expression in prostate is higher in the peripheral than in the transition zone," Cancer Lett 215 (2004): 69–78.

Prostate Specific Antigen

1 Olsson, A Y., et al., "Expression of prostate-specific antigen (PSA) and human glandular kallikrein 2 (hk2) in ileum and other extraprostatic tissues," Int J Cancer 113 (2005): 290–7.

2 De Lamirande, E., et al., "Semenogelin, the main protein of the human semen function, regulates sperm function," Semin Thromb Hemostat 33 (2007):60–8.

3 Bosch, J., et al., "Establishing normal reference ranges for PSA change with age in a population-based study: The Krimpen study," The Prostate 66 (2005): 335–43.

4   Catalona ,WJ., M.D., "PSA Velocity: Important New Tool in Fight Against Prostate Cancer," http://www.drcatalona. com/quest/Summer04/quest_summer04_2. asp (accessed Nov. 7, 2009).

5   Ibid.

6   Yu, H., et al., "Prostate-specific antigen in milk of lactating women," Clin Chem 41 (1995): 54–8.

7   Aksoy, Y., et al., "Serum insulin-like growth factor-1 and insulin-like growth factor binding protein-3 in localized, metastasized prostate cancer and benign prostatic hypertrophy," Urol Int 72 (2004):62–5.

8   Ibid.

9   Cohen, P., et al., "Biological effects of prostate specific antigen as an insulin-like growth factor binding protein-3 protease," J Endocrinol 142 (1994): 407–15.

10 Ibid.

11 Cohen, P., et al., "Prostate-specific antigen (PSA) is an insulin-like growth factor binding protein-3 protease found in seminal plasma," J Clin Endocrinol Metab 75 (1992): 1046–53.

12 Réhault, S., et al., "Insulin-like growth factor binding proteins (IGFBPs) as potential physiological substrates for human kallikreins hK2 and hK3," Eur J Biochem 268 (2001):2960–8.

13 Ibid.

14 Medscape "Ethnic Disparities in Breast Cancer: Incidence, Mortality & Stage,", http://www.medscape.com/viewarticle/566827_2 (accessed Nov. 7, 2009).

African-American Men and Prostate Cancer:

1   Rajbahu, K., et al., "Racial Origin is associated with poor awareness of prostate cancer in UK men, but can be increased by simple information," Prostate Cancer 10 (2007): 256–60.

2   ITZCARIBBEAN.COM 2009 "FOR THE CARIBBEAN COMMUNITY IN LONDON,", http://www.itzcaribbean.com/prostate_cancer_charity.php (accessed Nov. 7, 2009).

3   Winter, DL., et al., "Plasma levels of IGF-1, IGF-2 and IGFBP-3 in white and African-American men at increased risk of prostate cancer," Urology 58 (2001): 614–8.

4   Stattin, P., et al., "Plasma insulin-like growth factor-1, insulin-like growth factor–binding proteins, and prostate cancer risk: a prospective study," J Natl Cancer Inst 92 (2000): 1910–7.

5   Hernandez, W., et al., "IGF-1 and IGFBP-3 gene variants influence on serum levels and prostate cancer risk in African-Americans," Carcinogenesis 28 (2007): 2154–9.

6   Tricoli, JV., et al., "Racial differences in insulin-like growth factor binding protein-3 in men at increased risk of prostate cancer," Urology 54 (1999): 178–82.

7   Henderson, RJ., et al., "Prostate-specific antigen (PSA) and PSA density: racial differences in men without prostate cancer," J Natl Cancer Instit 89 (1997): 134–8.

8   Odedina, FT., et al., "Roots of prostate cancer in African-American men," J Natl Med Assoc 98 (2006): 539–43.

9   Garland, CF., et al., "The role of Vitamin D in cancer prevention," Am J Public Health 96 (2006): 252–61.

10   Ibid.

11   Chang, BL., et al., "Polymorphisms in the CYP1A1 gene are associated with prostate cancer risk," Int J Cancer 106 (2003):375–8.

12 Tang, YM., et al., "Human CYP1B1 Leu432Val gene polymorphism: ethnic distribution in Afircan-Americans, Caucasians and Chinese; oestradiol hydroxylase activity; and distribution in prostate cancer cases and controls," Pharmacogenetics 10 (2000): 761–6.

13 Ibid.

14 Scrimshaw, NS., et al., "The acceptability of milk and milk products in populations with a high prevalence of lactose intolerance." Am J Clin Nutr 48 (1988): 1079–159.

15 Suarez, FL., et al., "Tolerance to the daily ingestion of two cups of milk by individuals claiming lactose intolerance," Am J Clin Nutr 65 (1997): 1502–6.

16 Lactose Intolerance & Minorities 2008 "The Real Story," http://www.nationaldairycouncil.org/nationaldairycouncil/nutrition/lactose/lactoseIntolerance.pdf (accessed Nov.7, 2009).

Prostate Cancer: The Epigenetics

1   Seer Statistical Data Base U.S. Government,"Age Adjusted Incidence Rates by Race For Prostate Cancer, Ages 20–54, Males, Seer 9 Registries for 1974–2004, Age Adjusted to the 2000 Standard Population. (2008) http://www.seer.cancer.gov/ (accessed Nov.7,2009).

2   Seer Statistical Data Base U.S.
    Government."Prostate cancer
    incidence 1975–2004 for African-
    American men, Caucasian men, and
    all men," (2008) http://www.seer.
    cancer.gov/ (accessed Nov.7, 2009)

3   Schaid, DJ., et al., "Evidence for autosomal
    dominant inheritance of prostate cancer,"
    Am J Hum Genet 62 (1998): 1425–1438.

4   Daniel O'Sullivan. Figure Two: Mitosis
    (2008). Reproduced by permission.

5   Daniel O'Sullivan. Figure Three:
    DNA strand split during mitosis
    (2008) Reproduced by permission.

6   Daniel O'Sullivan. Figure Four:
    Two identical DNA strands (2008).
    Reproduced by permission.

7   Daniel O'Sullivan.Figure Five:
    Incorrect DNA match (2008).
    Reproduced by permission.

8   Diagram by Daniel O'Sullivan.
    Figure Six: Methyl group (2008).
    Reproduced by permission.

9   Daniel O'Sullivan. Figure Seven:
    CpG islands unmethylated (2008).
    Reproduced by permission.

10 Daniel O'Sullivan. Figure Eight:
    CpG islands methylated (2008).
    Reproduced by permission.

11 Fernández, PL., et al., "Alterations of cell cycle-regulatory genes in prostate cancer," Pathobiology 701 (2002) : 1–10.

12 Mhawech, P., et al., "Downregulation of 14–3–3sigma in ovary, prostate and endometrial carcinoma, is associated with CpG island methylation," Mod Pathol 18 (2005): 340–8.

13 Vardhman, K., et al., "Transgenerational inheritance of epigenetic states at the murine Axin allele occurs after maternal and paternal transmission," Proc Natl Acad Sci 100 (2003): 2538–2542.

14 Chung, W., et al., "Identification of novel tumor markers in prostate, colon and breast cancer by unbiased methylation profiling," PLoS ONE 3 (2008) e:2079.

15 Ibid.

16 Kang, GH., et al., "Aberrant CpG island hypermethylation of multiple genes in prostate cancer and prostatic intraepithelial neoplasia," J Pathol 202 (2004): 233–40.

17 Ellinger, J., et al., "CpG island hypermethylation at multiple gene sites in diagnosis and prognosis of prostate cancer,"Urology 71 (2008):161–7.

18 Nephew, KP., et al., "Epigenetic silencing in cancer initiation and progression," Cancer Lett 190 (2003): 125–33.

19 Söder, O. "Perinatal imprinting by estrogen and adult prostate disease," PNAS 102 (2005): 1269–70. www.pnas.org/cgi/doi/10.1073/pnas.0409703102 (accessed Nov. 7, 2009).

20 Ibid.

21 Omoto, Y., et al., "Estrogen receptor alpha and imprinting of the neonatal mouse ventral prostate,"Pro Natl Acad Sci. 102 (2005): 1484–9.

22 SEER Statistical Data Base. U.S. Government. (2008) "Prostate cancer incidence 1975–2004 for African-American men, Caucasian men, and all men," ,http://www.seer.cancer.gov/ (accessed Nov. 7, 2009).

23 Cavalieri, E., et al., "Catechol ortho-quinones: the electrophilic compounds that form depurinatin DNA adducts and could initiate cancer and other diseases," Carcinogenesis 23 (2002): 1071–77.

Modern Dairy Practices

1   Jang, W., et al., "Purification and Characterization of recombinant bovine growth hormone produced in Escherichia coli,"Biotech Letters. 20 (1998): 269–73.

2   Biotechnology Information Series (Bio-3)
    North Central Regional Extension
    Publication Iowa State University–
    University Extension 1993 "Bovine
    Somatotropin (bSt)," http://www.biotech.
    iastate.edu/biotech_info_series/Bovine_
    Somatotropin.html (accessed Nov. 7, 2009).

3   Smith J., Council for Responsible Genetics
    2004, "Whistleblowers, Threats and
    Bribes: A Short History of Genetically
    Engineered Bovine Growth Hormone,"
    http://www.councilforresponsiblegenetics.
    org/ViewPage.aspx?pageId=125
    (accessed Nov. 7, 2009).

4   Ibid.

5   Ibid.

6   Ibid.

7   Ibid.

8   Biotechnology Information Series (Bio-3)
    North Central Regional Extension
    Publication Iowa State University–
    University Extension 1993 "Bovine
    Somatotropin (bSt)," http://www.biotech.
    iastate.edu/biotech_info_series/Bovine_
    Somatotropin.html (accessed Nov. 7, 2009).

9   Nicholson, J., eHow™ How To Do
    Just About Anything. (2009) "Pros
    and Cons of rBGH," http://www.
    ehow.com/about_5542397_pros-cons-
    rbgh.html (accessed Nov. 7, 2009).

10 Miller M A. Dr. IPCS INCHEM Home, "Bovine Somatotropins First Draft,"(2008) http://www.inchem.org/documents/jecfa/jecmono/v31je08.htm (accessed Nov. 7, 2009).

11 Daxenberger, A., et al., "Increased milk levels of insulin-like growth factor 1 (IGF-1) for the identification of bovine somatotropin (bST) treated cows," Analyst 12 (1998): 2429–35.

12 Ibid.

13 Ibid.

14 Ibid.

15 Smith J., Council For Responsible Genetics 2004, "Whistleblowers, Threats and Bribes: A Short History of Genetically Engineered Bovine Growth Hormone," http://www.councilforresponsiblegenetics.org/ViewPage.aspx?pageId=125 (accessed Nov. 7, 2009).

16 Dr. Lyndom Larcom, e-mail message to author, January 6 2004.

17 Smith J., Council For Responsible Genetics 2004, "Whistleblowers, Threats and Bribes: A Short History of Genetically Engineered Bovine Growth Hormone," http://www.councilforresponsiblegenetics.org/ViewPage.aspx?pageId =125 (accessed Nov. 7, 2009).

18 Ganmaa, D., et al., "The possible role of female sex hormones in milk from pregnant cows in the development of breast, ovarian and corpus uteri cancers," Med Hypotheses 65 (2005): 1028–37.

19 Ganmaa, D., Harvard Gazette 2006 http://www.news.harvard. edu/gazette/2006/12.07/11-dairy. htmililiters (accessed Jan. 8, 2008).

20 Yalcin, A., "Emerging Therapeutic Potential of Whey Proteins and Peptides,"Curr Phar Des 12 (2006): 1637–43.

21 Skabar, A., About.Com., 2009 "Common Dairy-Derived Ingredients in Food Products," http://dairyfreecooking. about.com/od/dairyfreebasics/tp/ Dairy-Derived-Ingredient-List. htm (accessed Nov. 7, 2009).

22 Ibid.

23 Wolford, ST., et al., "Measurement of estrogens in cow's milk, human milk and dairy products," J DairySci 62 (1979):1458–63.

24 Sparks, AL., et al., "Insulin-like growth factor-1 and its binding proteins in colostrum compared to measures in serum of Holstein neonates," J DairySci 86 (2003): 2022–9.

Calcium from Dairy: The Myth

1   Feskanich, D., et al., "Milk, Dietary Calcium, and Bone Fractures in Women: A 12-Year Prospective Study,"Am J Public Health 87 (1997): 992–997.

2   Ibid.

3   Ibid.

4   Lanou, AJ., et al., "Calcium, dairy products, and bone health in children and young adults: a reevaluation of the evidence," Pediatrics 115 (2005): 736–43.

5   Ibid.

6   Sheikh, MS., et al., "Gastrointestinal absorption of calcium from milk and calcium salts," NE J Med 317 (1987): 532–536.

7   Zhao, Y., et al., "Calcium bioavailability of calcium carbonate fortified soymilk is equivalent to cow's milk in young women," J Nutr 135 (2005):2379–82.

8   "FDA nutrition label,"(2008) http://www.fda.gov/Food/LabelingNutrition/default.htm (accessed Nov. 7, 2009).

9   Ibid.

10 Ibid.

The American Grocery Cart: Your Toasted Cheese Sandwich

1 Little Miss Muffet Rhyme, 2009 "Nursery Rhyme & History," http://www.rhymes.org.uk/little_miss_muffet.htm (accessed Nov. 7, 2009).

2 Hakkak, R., et al., "Dietary whey protein protects against azoxymethane-induced colon tumors in male rats," Cancer Epidemiol Biomarkers Prev 10 (2001): 555–8.

3 Reverse Osmosis Milk, Whole Milk, 2006, "Preconcentration Ahead of Cheese Production," http://www.mssincorporated.com/reverseosmosis.htm (accessed Nov. 7, 2009).

4 Kaddouri, H., et al., "Microwave treatment modify antigenicity properties of bovine milk proteins," AfricanJ Biotechnology 5 (2006): 1267–70.

5 Hidalgo, J., et al., "Solubility and heat stability of whey protein concentrates," J DairySci 60 (1977): 1515–18.

6 U.S. Department of Health and Human Services, FDA, "Pasteurized Milk Ordinance 2007," (2008) http://www.fda.gov/default.htm (accessed Nov. 7, 2009).

7 Ibid.

8   Daxenberger, A., et al., "Increased milk levels of insulin-like growth factor 1 (IGF-1) for the identification of bovine somatotropin (bST) treated cows," Analyst 123 (1998): 2429–35.

9   Carpenter, K., eHow™, How To Do Just About Everything, "Does Whole Milk Contain Water?," (2009) http://www.ehow.com/way_5376805_whole-milk-contain-water.html (accessed Nov 15, 2009).

10   Grosvenor, C., et al., "Hormones and growth factors in milk," EndocrineReviews 14 (1993): 710–28.

11   Wolford, S.T., et al., "Measurement of estrogens in cow's Milk, human milk, and dairyproducts," J Dairy Sci 62 (1979):1458–63.

12   McGuigan, B., wiseGeek™ , 2009 "What is Casein?)," http://www.wisegeek.com/what-is-casein.htm (accessed Nov.7, 2009).

13   Ibid.

14   Wolford, S.T., et al., "Measurement of estrogens in cow's milk, human milk, and dairyproducts," J Dairy Sci 62 (1979): 1458–63.

15   U.S. Department of Agriculture, Economic Research Service, "U.S. Per Capita Food Avaliablity Dairy," (2007) http://www.ers.usda.gov/Search/?qt=Per%20Capita%20Milk%20Over%20time (accessed Nov. 7, 2009).

16 U.S. Department of Agriculture, Economic Research Service, "U.S. Per Capita Food Avaliablity Dairy," (2007) http://www.ers.usda.gov/Search/?qt=per+capita+cheese+over+time (accessed Nov. 7, 2009)

17 Hutchings, J., et al., "Metabolic Changes Produced By Human Growth Hormone (LI) In A Pituitary Dwarf," J Clin Endo &Metab 19 (1959): 759–69.

Is Anybody Listening?

1 Copy of biopsy report given to author by patient. (2008). Reproduced by permission.

2 Ibid.

3 Ibid.

4 Ibid.

5 Seeram, NP., et al., "Pomegranate ellagitannin-derived metabolites inhibit prostate cancer growth an localize to the mouse prostate gland," J Agric FoodChem 55 (2007): 7732–7

Hope

1 Marchione, M., ABC News, 2008 "Older men with prostate cancer can wait and see," http://www.abcnews.go.com/print?id=4281872 (accessed Nov. 7, 2009).

2 Ibid.

3   Sakr,WA., et al., "Epidemiology of high grade prostatic intraepithelial neoplasia," Pathol Res Pract 191 (1995):838–41.

4   Whiteside, M., et al., Developed by the Office of Cancer Surveillance in support of the Tennessee Comprehensive Cancer Control Coalition (TCCCC) "Burden of Cancer in Tennessee. Tennessee Comprehensive Cancer Control Program Report," 2007:16, http://health.stste.tn.us/Downloads/TnBurdenofCancer08.pdf. (accessed June 8, 2008).

5   Ibid.

6   Ibid.

Epilogue

1   Hemminki, K., et al., "Familial association of prostate cancer with other cancers in the Swedish Family-Cancer Database," Prostate 65 (2005): 188–94.

2   Pastural, E., et al., "RIZ1 repression is associated with insulin-like factor-1 signaling activation in chronic myeloid leukemia cell lines," Oncogene 26 (2007):1586–94.

3   Harris W. M.D. "Cancer and the Vegetarian Diet," 1999 http://www.vegsource.com/harris/cancer_vegdiet.htm (accessed Feb 8, 2008).

4   Pastural, E., et al., "RIZ1 repression is associated with insulin-like factor-1 signaling activation in chronic myeloid leukemia cell lines," Oncogene 26 (2007):1586–94.

5   Harris W. M.D. "Cancer and the Vegetarian Diet," 1999 http://www.vegsource.com/harris/cancer_vegdiet.htm (accessed Feb. 8, 2008).

6   Shames, D., et al., "A Genome-Wide Screen for Promoter Methylation in Lung Cancer Identifies Novel Methylation Markers for Multiple Malignancies," PLOS ONE, 12 (2006):http://www.ncbi.nlm.nih.gov/pmc/articles/PMC1716188/ (accessed Nov. 8, 2009).

7   Ibid.

Appendix A

1   Chung, W., et al., "Identification of Novel Tumor Markers in Prostate., Colon, and Breast Cancer by Unbiased Methylation Profiling," PLoS ONE (2008):2079, http:// www.plosone.org (accessed Nov. 8, 2009).

Appendix B

1   infoplease® Pearson Education
    2000–2009 " Per Capita Consumption
    of Principal Foods," http://www.
    infoplease.com/ipa/A0104742.
    htmililiters (accessed Nov 8, 2009).

2   Filippone P., About.com©: Home
    Cooking, "Ground Beef Labels,"
    http://homecooking.about.com/od/
    beef/a/groundbeeflabel.htmililiters
    (accessed Nov. 8, 2009).

3   Filippone P.,About.com©: Home
    Cooking, 2009 "Ground Beef
    Labels," http://homecooking.about.
    com/od/beef/a/groundbeeflabel.
    htmililiters (accessed Nov. 8, 2009).

Appendix C

1   United States Department of
    Agriculture National Agricultural
    Statistics Service, "DairyProducts
    2005 Summary,", http://www.nass.
    usda.gov/ (accessed Nov. 8, 2009).

2   Producer-Handler Records of Production,
    "Weighing, Testing and Utilization,",
    http://arcweb.sos.state.or.us/rules/
    OARS_600/OAR_603/603_067.
    htmililiters (accessed Nov. 8, 2009).

3   U.S. Census Bureau 2005, "National and State Population Estimates,", http://www.census.gov/popest/states/NST-ann-est2005.html (accessed Nov. 8, 2009).

4   Malekinejad, H., et al., "Naturally occurring estrogens in processed and raw milk (from gestated cows)," Journal Agric FoodChemistry 54 (2006): 9785–91.

Appendix D

1   Wolford, ST., et al., "Measurement of estrogens in cow's milk, human milk and dairy products," Journal of Dairyn Science 62 (1979): 1458–63.

2   Narenden, R., et al., "Hormonal induction of lactation: estrogen and progesterone in milk,"Journal of DairyScience 62 (1979): 1069–75.

3   Pape-Zambito, DA., et al., "Concentrations of 17-estradiol in Holstein whole milk," Journal of Dairy Science 90 (2007): 3308–13.

4   Daxenberger, A., et al., "Possible health impact of animal estrogens in food," Human Reproduction Update 7 (2001):340–55.

Appendix E

1 United States Government SEER Statistical Data Base, Division of Cancer Control
   and Population Sciences, National Cancer
   Institute, "Cancer Incidence Rates for
   Men, 1975–2002," (2005):http://www.
   nass.usda.gov/ (accessed Nov. 8, 2009).

APPENDIX A: HEAT MAPS

The following heat maps *B*, *C*, and *D* show the degree of methylation ("turn off") of various suppressor genes in the cancers outlined above. The numbers vertically are the patient biopsy specimen numbers. The letter-number combinations listed horizontally are the specific suppressor genes analyzed. In figure *A*, the commercially available cancer tissue cultures are designated horizontally, and the specific suppressor genes are listed vertically.

It is interesting to note that there are a significant number of the same genes methylated (turned off) in each of these tumors.

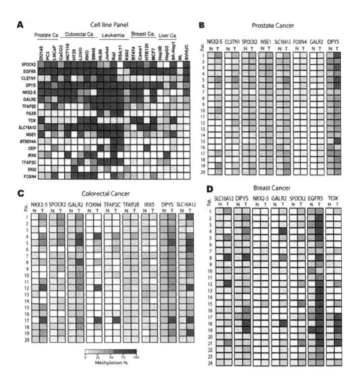

Source: Chung, W., et al., "Identification of Novel Tumor Markers in Prostate, Colon, and Breast Cancer by Unbiased MethylationProfiling," *PLoS ONE* (2008):2079, http:// www.plosone.org (accessed Nov. 8, 2009). (Note: Normally the heat maps would be in colors of white to red. The original red was formatted to grayscale for the printing of this book.)

APPENDIX B:

Calculation of the Estimated Total Amount of Estrogens Consumed Daily from Beef

The cited average daily beef consumption per person is 62.9 pounds per year.[1] Conversion to grams per day: 62.9 pounds per person divided by 2.2 pounds per kilogram and multiplied by 1000 grams per kilogram equals 28,591 grams and divided by 365 days per year equals:

> 62.9 / 2.2 x 1000 / 365 = 78.4 grams of beef per person per day.

From cited literature, the average percent of beef that is fat is 11 percent.[2] This means there would be 78.4 multiplied by 11 percent equals:

78.4 x .011 = 8.6 grams of fat per person per day, and the remaining is muscle, or 69.8 grams of muscle per person per day.

Additional cited literature reveals that the average tallow consumption per person per year is 4.7 pounds, or 5.9 grams per person per day.[3]

Adding fat from beef and additional tallow gives us:

+ 5.9 = 14.5 grams of fat per person per day, and from above we have 69.8 grams of muscle per person per day.

If we use the residual estrogen values calculated by Hendrix and listed in the chapter on estrogens, we would have a total estrogen value for muscle of 70.28 picograms of estrone and 13.2 picograms of 17ß-estradiol, bringing the total estrogen residual in beef total to 83.5 picograms per gram of muscle. With this value, the total estrogen consumed daily from beef as muscle would be 69.8 grams of muscle per day multiplied by 83.5 picograms per gram of muscle to give total estrogen intake from muscle:

69.8 x 83.5 = 5828 picograms, or 5.8 nanograms.

For fat, we have a total of 14.5 grams of fat per person, per day from beef.

The total estrogen residue value by Hendrix for fat is 709.5 picograms of estrone and 30.4 picograms of

17ß-estradiol to give a total of 731 picograms of estrogens per person, per day, per gram of fat from beef.

This gives us 731 picograms of estrogen x 14.5 grams of fat, or 10,600 picgrams, or 10.6 nanograms of estrogen from fat. This gives us 10.6 (fat) + 5.8 (muscle) or 16.4 *nanograms of total estrogen from daily beef consumption.*

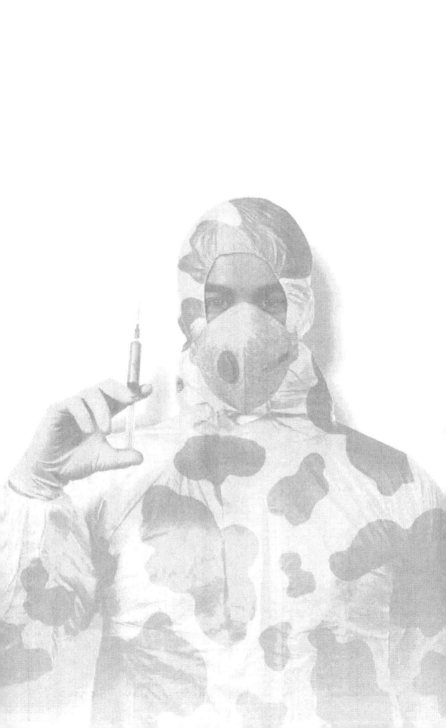

APPENDIX C:

Calculation of the Estrogen Content in a Typical Dairy Diet

From *Shultz and DairyProducts Profile*, we know that 169 billion pounds of dairy was marketed in 2005. Schultz also tells us that 62 percent was converted into milk and milk-derived products.[1]

In this calculation, I made an assumption that 50 percent of marketed products are consumed. This could be a conservative estimate.

There are 8.6 pounds per gallon of milk on average.[2] This would mean we have:

176,000,000,000 pounds of milk / 8.6 pounds per gallon = 20.44 billion gallons of milk produced per year.

The U.S. population was estimated at 293 million in 2005.[3] This would mean the gallons-per-person consumed equals:

20,440,000,000 / 293,000,000 = 70 gallons per person per year, or 70 / 365 = 0.19 gallons per person, per day, or 0.75 quarts or 719 milliliters of milk per person per day.

The average estrogen content was determined by averageing the totals for each estrogen in milk from Table Two in the Estrogen chapter. I intentionally left out the values for oleoyl estrone.

Now armed with the knowledge that the average consumption of milk on a daily basis is 719 milliliters per person per day, we will have a total estrogen intake per person per day of:

719 milliliters per day x 428 picograms per milliliters = 0.31 micrograms per day of total estrogen intake. Note: This does not include the values for the oleoyl-estrone that we talked about in the estrogen chapter. The values using oleoyl-estrone are much higher as I had discussed in the estrogen chapter.

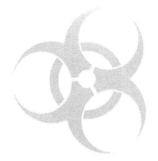

APPENDIX D:

Regression Analyses Graphs for
Comparison of Dairy Consumption
Related to Prostate, Ovarian,
And Lymphoma Cancers

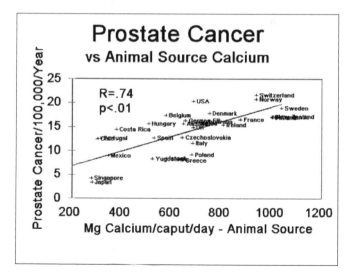

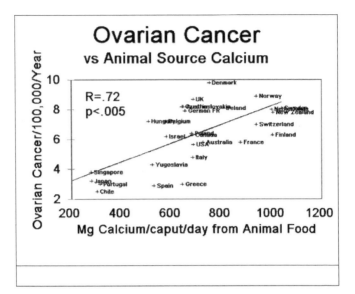

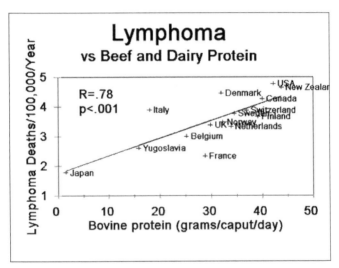

Source: Harris, W. MD, "Cancer and the Vegetarian Diet,"(1999) http://www.vegsource.com/harris/cancer_vegdiet.htm (accessed Feb. 8, 2008).

Note: William Harris, MD, is medical director of the Kaiser-Permanente Vegan Lifestyle Clinic (VLC) in Honolulu, Hawaii.

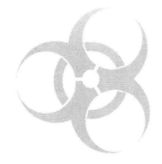

APPENDIX E:

Best Line Fit Development for Prostate
Cancer Incidence Versus Time Prior To 1975

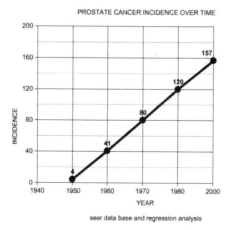

Source: This graph is a regression analysis of the best fit for the data
from the SEER United States Government SEER Statistical Data
Base, Division of Cancer Control and Population Sciences, National
Cancer Institute, "Cancer Incidence Rates for Men, 1975–2002,"
(2005):http://www.nass.usda.gov/.[1]

I have excluded data points between the years 1986 and 1995 because the data points between these years were artificially inflated because the newer PSA test became available. The PSA analysis detected cancers not picked up by digital exam. The incidence numbers after 1995 then reflected the actual incidence then determined by PSA. The slopes of the incidence line prior to use of PSA and after PSA are curiously similar. It is observed that the incidence line strikes zero on the timeline at around 1948.

APPENDIX F:

Alternative Protein Sources

Bee Pollen Granules, http://www.bulkfoods.com—Bee pollen contains around 50 percent protein, much of which is in the form of free amino acids. It is also high in the B-complex vitamins and enzymes.

Unflavored Gelatine, nutritional supplement, www.bulkfoods.com—Gelatin (Gelatine) is made from the collagen protein found in bone, skin, and cartilage. When beef or pork is boiled, the collagen is extracted and changes into gelatin. Our gelatin is an excellent source of protein containing over 85 percent protein. Typical usage: 4 teaspoons per day. May be mixed in noncarbonated juices or with foods.

Brown Rice/Rice Protein, www.bulkfoods.com—contains 80 percent protein. Rice protein concentrate is made from non-GMO sprouted brown rice grains. The amino acid profile is approximately 98 percent similar to mother's milk. A vegan, hypoallergenic, natural-grain protein concentrate. Has a strong flavor profile, as some of the protein is in free amino acids.

Organic Hemp Protein Powder

www.evitaminstore.com—Imagine an organic food with 37 percent protein, 10 percent beneficial fats, 43 percent fiber (90 percent soluble, 10 percent insoluble), chlorophyll, magnesium, zinc, and iron. Sound too good to be true? It's not—hempseed is one of nature's most perfect superfoods. Nutiva's delicious Organic Hemp Protein Powder is:

- USDA organic
- 54 percent + RDI of Fiber
- A delicious high-fiber protein drink mix!

Extremely nutritious

One serving provides 11 grams of raw, organic protein and a whopping 14 grams of fiber (54 percent of the RDI). Hemp contains all 8 essential amino acids with the bonus of good-for-you essential fatty acids.

Organic Blue-Green Algae Powder, www.mynatu-ralmarket.com—This rare superfood is a protein power-house. It provides a highly bio available protein that is 80 percent assimilated in our bodies (compared to meat protein, which is 20 percent assimilated), and its amino acid profile is optimal for humans. Klamath Lake algae is also the world's most concentrated source of chlo-rophyll, a valuable phytonutrient considered by many to be one of nature's most cleansing and regenerating substances.

www.bodybuilding.com

SciVation Xtend—Xtend is a precise, scientific blend of energy aminos consisting of the proven 2:1:1 ratio of branched chain amino acids (L-Leucine, L-Isoleucine, and L-Valine), Glutamine, Citrulline Malate, and Vitamin B6 that will give you the energy you need to maximize your training while enhanc-ing recovery at the same time. The advanced compo-nents in Xtend have been scientifically proven to help:

- Speed recovery
- Enhance ATP production and promote cell volumization
- Decrease muscle breakdown and cortisol levels
- Avoid fatigue by blocking entry of fatigue-inducing tryptophan into the brain
- Increase protein synthesis, immune func-tion, and digestive health

- Promote vasodilation, which can lead to better assimilation and absorption of protein

- Elevate growth hormone levels

www.bodybuilding.com

Note: Appendix F was prepared by Mr. Paul Eastwood, a professional trainer, who lives in Wilmington, North Carolina. Paul can be contacted at: paulpauleastwoodonline.com

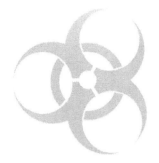

APPENDIX G:

Compound Interest Curve Demonstrating Effect of Accumulating Interest

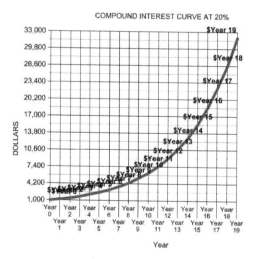

The interest curve above is a demonstration of what happens in successive years when something is accumulating. In this case it is dollars earned from interest at 20 percent per year.

Let us replace interest with suppressor genes being turned off and passed on to subsequent generations. The x-axis would then be incidence. Does this curve look familiar to you? It should because it is identical to the curve we see for incidence of prostate cancer over time in black and white men. It would be steeper for black men because they have higher levels of IGF-1 and are turning off more suppressor genes per generation.

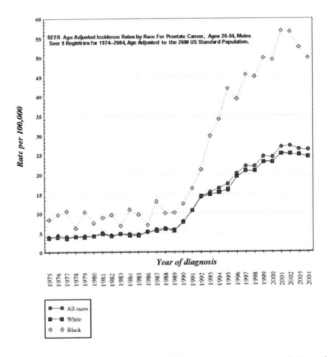

Source: Seer Statistical Data Base U.S. Government," Age Adjusted Incidence Rates by Race For Prostate Cancer, Ages 20–54, Males, Seer 9 Registries for 1974–2004, Age Adjusted to the 2000 Standard Population., http://www.seer.cancer.gov/ (accessed Nov.7, 2009).

APPENDIX H:

Alternative Substitutes for Certain Dairy Products

Substitutes for milk include:

1. Soy silk milk. It comes in different flavors.

2. Rice Dream™. This is a rice-based milk substitute. It is a little on the sweet side.

3. Almond milk. It is delicious but can be costly.

Substitutes for butter include:

1. Benecol™ Tastes like butter but best not to fry or bake with.
2. Earth Balance™ margarine.

Substitutes for cheese include:

1. Follow Your Heart Vegan Gourmet® Cheeses.

Substitutes for cream cheese and sour cream:

1. Toffuti.

Substitutes for yogurt include:

1. So Nice Dairy Free Yogurt®.
2. Silk® Cultured Soy Yogurt.

There are many great resources on the Internet where you can find dairy-free products. One of the great Web sites is: http://www.godairyfree.org/Food-to-Eat/Shopping-List/Non-Dairy-Alternatives-Sour-Cream-Whipped-Cream-Yogurt-Tofu.htmililiters

APPENDIX I: LIST OF ILLUSTRATIONS AND TABLES

Prostate Cancer: The Disease

1. Figure One: Male reproductive tract
2. Figure Two: Normal prostate tissue
3. Figure Three: Normal p53 mediated cell death
4. Figure Four: Defective p53 and cancer colony

Prostate Cancer: The Statistics

(PIN) by autopsy, ethnic group, and age from various countries

Prostate Cancer: Food Association Studies

1. Figure One: Ovarian cancer incidence by country versus animal source calcium
2. Figure Two: Prostate cancer incidence by country versus animal source calcium

Harry Steenbock and The Antirachitic Machine

1. Figure One: Conversion of ergosterol to vitamin D2 by ultraviolet light
2. Figure Two: Dr. Steenbock and his Antirachitic Machine
3. Figure Three: Segment of the Steenbock patent
4. Figure Four: Folded protein
5. Figure Five: Ultraviolet light denaturing a protein
6. Figure Six: SEER incidence rates of cancer for men, 1975–2002

Insulin-like Growth Factor One: The Killer

1. Table One: IGF-1 and estrogen interactions after ingestion of dairy products

Estrogens: The Accomplice

2. Figure One: Estratriol

3. Figure Two: Estradiol

4. Figure Three: Estrone

5. Figure Four: Conversion of estrone and testosterone to 17 betaestradiol as occurs in the prostate gland

6. Table One: Estrogenresidues in beef expressed in picograms per gram of each tissue by Hendricks, 1983

7. Table Two: Type of estrogen found in milk and author (Values are in picograms per milliliter)

8. Table Four: Relative binding capacities of estrogens and estrogen metabolites and other chemicals to estrogen receptors alpha and beta

Prostate Specific Antigen

1. Table One: PSA effect on IGF-1 and end result

African-American Men on Dairy in the U.S.: Multiple Jeopardies

1. Figure One: Prostate cancer incidence 1975–2004 for black men, white men, and all men

2. Table One: Prostate cancer incidence north-south gradient comparison table

3. Table Two: Biologic process and effect versus ethnicity

4. Table Three: Non-Westernized African country prostate cancer incidence

Prostate Cancer: The Epigenetics

1. Figure One: Prostate cancer incidence 1975- 2004 for African-American men, Caucasian men, and all men

2. Figure Two: Mitosis

3. Figure Three: DNA strand split during mitosis

4. Figure Four: Two identical strands of DNA

5. Figure Five: Incorrect DNA match

6. Figure Six : Methyl group

7. Figure Seven: CpG islands unmethylated

8. Figure Eight: CpG islands methylated

9. Figure Nine: Prostate cancer heat map

Modern Dairy Practices

1. Figure One: Normal distribution curves for IGF-1 in milk from cows given rBGH versus cows not given rBGH

Calcium from Dairy: The Myth

1. Table One: Calcium intake recommendation versus age

2. Table Two: Recommended calcium intake for adults

3. Table Three: Various foods and calcium content

4. Figure One: FDA nutrition label

The American Grocery Cart: Your Toasted Cheese Sandwich

1. Table One: Pasteurization and FDA guidelines

2. Figure One: Pounds per capita whole milk over time

3. Figure Two: Pounds per capita cheese over time

Is Anybody Listening?

1. Figure One: prostate biopsy one year before start of dairy-free diet

2. Figure Two: Patient prostate biopsy one year after a dairy-free diet

An Epidemic

1. Table One: Genetic linkage events in prostate cancers

2. Table Two: Cancers and their respective methylated genes versus benign tissue methylation of these genes

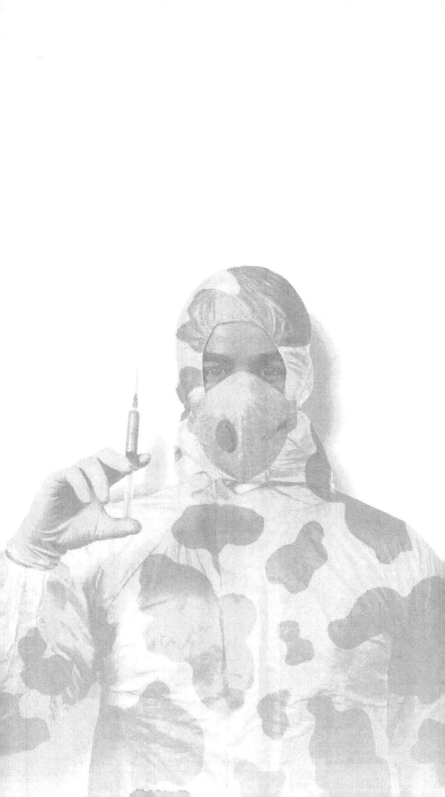

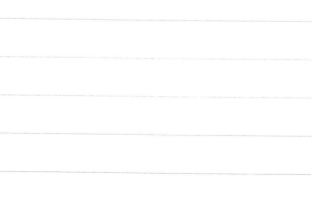

READER'S NOTES

ROBERT BIBB, MD

ROBERT BIBB, MD

Made in the USA
Middletown, DE
01 November 2015